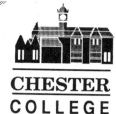

World Health Organization
Geneva 1989

ISBN 92 4 154242 X

TYPESET IN INDIA

PRINTED IN ENGLAND

87/7454—Macmillan/Clays—7000

Contents

Introduction

Volume 1 of the *Lexicon of psychiatric and mental health terms* is designed for use in conjunction with Chapter V (Mental disorders) of the ninth revision of the *International classification of diseases* (ICD-9). The lexicon is a step towards the development of an international nomenclature of mental disorders as part of the *International Nomenclature of Diseases* (IND).[1] Many of the terms defined in this volume will be used, as far as possible, in the tenth revision of the ICD (ICD-10).

The work to develop this lexicon has been partly an element of a joint project on diagnosis and classification of mental disorders and alcohol- and drug-related problems, co-sponsored by WHO and the US Alcohol, Drug Abuse, and Mental Health Administration (ADAMHA). Preparation of this first volume was recommended by a WHO/ADAMHA Scientific Working Group that met in April 1981 in Mannheim under the chairmanship of Professor E. Strömgren.

Relationship to ICD-9

This volume contains definitions of over 300 terms that appear in Chapter V of ICD-9, either as numbered diagnostic rubrics, already provided with glossary notes, or as inclusion or descriptive terms without definitions. For 125 terms, definitions are reproduced, with certain modifications, from the glossary in Chapter V of ICD-9, or other WHO sources. The remaining definitions have been prepared *de novo*.

Chapter V is the only section of ICD-9 that has a glossary. This glossary of mental disorders, prepared by an international group of experts for use with ICD-8, aims 'not to impose theoretical concepts upon users ... but simply to guide them in classifying mental disorders for purposes of international coding and communication with others'.

The ICD-9 glossary has proved valuable, but experience in its use has shown the need to enlarge and supplement the material, which is confined to the principal categories of disease, and contains references to a variety of psychopathological concepts that are not themselves defined.

The WHO/ADAMHA Working Group identified, as a first priority, the need to tackle the terms in the ICD-9 glossary that called for further elaboration. By providing tentative definitions of these terms, and some additional ones, this publication complements the ICD-9 glossary.

---

[1] The IND is a joint project of the Council for International Organizations of Medical Sciences and the World Health Organization, which aims to provide a single recommended name for every morbid entity.

Drafting of definitions

Definitions were drafted by a small task force consisting of Professor M. Shepherd, Professor E. Strömgren, Professor E. Essen-Möller, and Dr A. Jablensky (WHO Project Coordinator), assisted by Dr J. Gallagher. The rules established for the *International nomenclature of diseases* (IND), and set forth in guidelines approved by the IND Technical Steering Committee, were followed as far as the current state of the 'common language' of psychiatry allowed. The draft definitions were circulated for comments to members of the WHO Expert Advisory Panel on Mental Health, the International Advisory Group of the Joint Project on Diagnosis and Classification of Mental Disorders and Alcohol- and Drug-related Problems, and other experts in various parts of the world, representing all the major schools of psychiatry.[1]

The comments and suggestions were reviewed, and editorial changes incorporated into the text, by Professor M. Shepherd and Dr A. Jablensky.

For definitions originating in ICD-9, or other WHO sources, the following symbols are given in square brackets at the end of the quotation:

[MDG] = *Mental disorders. Glossary and guide to their classification in accordance with the ninth revision of the International classification of diseases.* Geneva, World Health Organization, 1978.

[ARD] = Edwards, G. et al., ed. *Alcohol-related disabilities.* Geneva, World Health Organization, 1977 (WHO Offset Publication, No. 32).

[DE] = Gastaut, H. (in collaboration with an international group of experts). *Dictionary of epilepsy. Part I. Definitions.* Geneva, World Health Organization, 1973.

How to use the lexicon

This volume is in three parts, corresponding to the three broad categories into which the technical terms of Chapter V of ICD-9 can be classified.

Part I — Names of diseases, syndromes, and other conditions or disorders that appear as diagnoses in psychiatry.

Part II — Names of symptoms or signs of disorders and other psychopathological terms used in the description or definition of various diseases, syndromes and conditions.

---

[1] A list of the people who made comments and suggestions, or helped in any way in the preparation of the manuscript, is given on page 66.

Part III — Terms for more abstract concepts that are used in the delimitation of major classes or categories of disorders, or that concern general rules and principles of classification of psychiatric conditions.

Alphabetical arrangement

An alphabetical arrangement has been chosen for each of the three parts, instead of following the current ICD-9 numerical sequence of rubrics, or attempting a thesaurus-like grouping of terms.

The entry word chosen for each composite term is the one that, in the judgement of the editors, is most likely to be used by the reader as an 'identifier' of a concept, or group of related concepts. For example, dementia was thought to be a convenient entry word for **presenile dementia** and **senile dementia**, but epileptic was considered a more appropriate entry word for **epileptic dementia** because it allowed the grouping of the latter concept with the closely related ones of **epileptic psychosis**, acute and chronic.

Entries

The code number of the ICD-9 rubric in which the term appears is given in brackets after each entry. For most of the terms, existing synonyms (or near synonyms) have been listed. The note 'deprecated' follows any term or synonym that should no longer be used.

Where it is recommended that the user consults a related term, there is the suggestion to 'See also: ... '. Some definitions include a historical or general comment that cannot be classed as part of the definition itself. These are listed under 'Comment: ...'.

Index

An alphabetical index of all entries and synonyms is given on page 69.

Acknowledgements

The preparation of this volume of the lexicon was supported partly by funds provided through the WHO/ADAMHA Joint Project on Diagnosis and Classification of Mental Disorders and Alcohol- and Drug-related Problems, and partly by funds provided by CIOMS through the joint CIOMS/WHO programme for the International Nomenclature of Diseases. These funds were granted to CIOMS by the Kuwait Foundation for the Advancement of Sciences and the Kuwait Ministry of Public Health.

Part I

Terms used in psychiatric diagnosis

Names of diseases, syndromes, and other conditions or disorders that appear as diagnoses in psychiatry

acute infective psychosis (ICD: 293.0) An acute, usually **confusional**, psychosis associated with infectious or parasitic disease.
See also: **symptomatic psychosis.**

acute reaction to stress (ICD: 308) Very transient disorders of any severity and nature which occur in individuals without any apparent pre-existing mental disorder in response to exceptional physical or mental **stress**, such as natural catastrophe or battle, and which usually subside within hours or days [MDG]. The acute reaction to stress may manifest a predominant disturbance of emotions, e.g., **panic states**, excitability, **fear, depression** or **anxiety**; a predominant disturbance of consciousness, e.g., **fugue**; or a predominant **psychomotor disturbance**, e.g., agitation or stupor.
Synonyms: catastrophic stress reaction; exhaustion delirium (deprecated); combat fatigue; post-traumatic stress disorder.

addiction (ICD: 303, 304) Surrender and devotion to the regular use of a medicinal or pleasurable substance for the sake of the relief, comfort, stimulation, or exhilaration that it affords; often with craving when the drug is absent, in addiction to opiates, barbiturates and morphine-like drugs, and perhaps in addiction to alcohol, cocaine, marijuana and amphetamine; together with apparently physical dependence in addiction to opiates and morphine-like analgesics, barbiturates, and possibly alcohol; together with increased tolerance (or adaptation) to opiates and morphine-like analgesics, barbiturates, and perhaps amphetamine and alcohol; and usually with psychotoxic effects during withdrawal in addiction to opiates, morphine-like analgesics, barbiturates and alcohol [ARD]. ICD-9 has expressed a preference for the replacement of the term 'addiction' by 'dependence'.
Synonym: substance dependence.

adjustment reaction (ICD: 309) Mild and transient disorders lasting longer than **acute reactions** to **stress**, which occur in individuals of any age without apparent pre-existing mental disorder. Such disorders are often relatively circumscribed or situation-specific, are generally reversible, and usually last only a few months. They are usually closely related in time and content to **stresses** such as bereavement, migration or separation experiences. Reactions to major stress that last longer than a few days are also included here. In children such disorders are associated with no significant distortion of development [MDG].

adjustment reaction with mixed disturbance of emotions and conduct (ICD: 309.4) Disorder fulfilling the general definition of adjustment reactions in which both emotional disturbance, and disturbance of conduct are prominent features [MDG].

adjustment reaction with predominant disturbance of conduct (ICD: 309.3) Mild or transient disorder, fulfilling the general criteria for **adjustment reaction**, in which the main disturbance involves conduct. For example, an adolescent grief reaction resulting in aggressive or antisocial disorder would be included here [MDG].

affective psychoses (ICD: 296) Mental disorders, usually recurrent, in which there is a severe disturbance of **mood** (mostly compounded of **depression** and **anxiety** but also manifested as **elation** and excitement) which is accompanied by one or more of the following: **delusions**, **perplexity**, disturbed attitude to self, disorder of perception and behaviour; these are all in keeping with the patient's prevailing mood (as are hallucinations when they occur). There is a strong tendency to suicide. For practical reasons, mild disorders of mood may also be included here if the symptoms match closely the descriptions given; this applies particularly to mild hypomania [MDG].
See also: bipolar disorder; depression; manic-depressive psychoses; de-
       pression, unipolar (monopolar); mania, unipolar (monopolar).

agoraphobia (ICD: 300.2) In current usage, abnormally intense dread of going out alone and of being in situations where there are many other people.
Comment: The condition was first described by Westphal in 1872 as a morbid
       fear of large open spaces.

alcohol abuse, nondependent (ICD: 305.0) Noxious consumption of alcohol, including acute alcohol intoxication and 'hangover' effects [MDG], but without the other features of the **alcohol dependence syndrome**.
Synonyms: inebriety; drunkenness.

alcohol dependence syndrome (ICD: 303) A state, psychic and usually also physical, resulting from taking alcohol, characterized by behavioural and other responses that always include a **compulsion** to take alcohol on a continuous or periodic basis in order to experience its psychic effects, and sometimes to avoid the discomfort of its absence; tolerance may or may not be present. A person may be dependent on alcohol and other drugs [MDG]. Dependence may be associated with **alcoholic psychosis** or with physical complications.
Synonyms: alcoholism (deprecated); chronic alcoholism (deprecated).

alcohol withdrawal syndrome (ICD: 291.8) A complex of symptoms ranging from hangover to **delirium tremens**, often occurring in severe forms when alcohol intake is stopped after a prolonged bout, sometimes beginning when the blood alcohol concentration is allowed to decline during a bout, and

sometimes manifested in mild forms after a brief session of heavy alcohol intake or a single intake of a large quantity of alcohol. The symptoms may include tremulousness, psychomotor and autonomic overactivity, gastric distress, headache, fever, sweating, hypertension, hyper-reflexia, nystagmus, seizures and **hallucinations** [ARD].
Synonym: abstinence syndrome.

alcoholic dementia (ICD: 291.2) Nonhallucinatory **dementia** occurring in association with the **alcohol dependence syndrome** but not characterized by the features of either **delirium tremens** or **Korsakov's psychosis** [MDG].
Synonyms: chronic alcoholic brain syndrome (deprecated); dementia associated with alcoholism (deprecated).

alcoholic hallucinosis (ICD: 291.3) A psychotic disorder usually of less than six months' duration, with slight or no **clouding of consciousness** and much anxious restlessness in which auditory **hallucinations**, mostly of voices uttering insults and threats, predominate [MDG].

alcoholic jealousy (ICD: 291.5) Chronic **paranoid** psychosis characterized by delusional **morbid jealousy** and associated with the **alcohol dependence syndrome** [MDG].
Synonyms: alcoholic paranoia; paranoid state in an alcohol-dependent person.

alcoholic psychoses (ICD: 291) Organic psychotic states due mainly to excessive consumption of alcohol; defects of nutrition are thought to play an important role. In some of these states, withdrawal of alcohol can be of etiological significance [MDG].

alcoholism (ICD: 303) (deprecated) In view of the loss of precision in usage of the term 'alcoholism', and its confusion with 'problem drinking' and other behaviours not definable as addictive or dependent, the term **alcohol dependence syndrome** is to be preferred in diagnostic usage and to define a disease.
Synonyms: alcohol dependence syndrome; chronic alcoholism (deprecated).

Alzheimer's disease (ICD: 290.1, 331.0) A primary degenerative polioencephalopathy of unknown etiology and pathogenesis, characterized morphologically by cortical atrophy with neurofibrillary tangles and senile plaques, with onset usually in the presenium or early senium. The course is progressive, leading terminally to profound dementia. The boundaries of the disease and its relation to other dementing conditions are still unclear.
See also: senile dementia, simple type, and presenile dementia.
Comment: The condition was first described by Alzheimer (1864-1915).
Synonym: morbus Alzheimer.

animal phobia (ICD: 300.2) A morbid fear of animals, most commonly small animals, e.g. mice and spiders.
Synonym: zoophobia.

anorexia nervosa (ICD: 307.1) A disorder in which the main features are persistent active refusal to eat and marked loss of weight. The level of activity and alertness is characteristically high in relation to the degree of emaciation. Typically the disorder begins in teenage girls but it may sometimes begin before puberty. Amenorrhoea is usual and there may be a variety of other physiological changes including slow pulse and respiration, low body temperature and dependent oedema. Unusual eating habits and attitudes towards food are typical and sometimes starvation follows or alternates with periods of overeating (see also bulimia). The accompanying psychiatric symptoms are diverse. Occasionally the disorder occurs in males [MDG].
Synonym: mental anorexia (deprecated).

anxiety hysteria (ICD: 300.2) (deprecated) A psychoanalytical concept introduced by Freud to describe a form of **hysteria** in which **anxiety** is manifest as a **phobic state**. The term has also been used for conditions characterized by a mixture of anxiety and **conversion** symptoms.

anxiety states (ICD: 300.0) Various combinations of physical and mental manifestations of **anxiety** not attributable to real danger and occurring either in attacks or as a persisting state. The anxiety is usually diffuse and may extend to **panic**. Other neurotic features such as obsessional or hysterical symptoms may be present but do not dominate the clinical picture [MDG].
Synonyms: anxiety neurosis; anxiety reaction.

arithmetical retardation, specific (ICD: 315.1) Disorders in which the main feature is serious impairment in the development of arithmetical **skills** which is not explicable in terms of general **mental retardation** or of inadequate schooling [MDG].
Synonyms: dyscalculia; developmental arithmetic disorder.

autism, infantile (ICD: 299.0) A rare syndrome that in most cases is present from birth or begins in the first 30 months. Responses to auditory and sometimes to visual stimuli are abnormal and there are usually severe problems in the understanding of spoken language. Speech is delayed and, if it develops, is characterized by **echolalia**, the reversal of pronouns, immature grammatical structure, and inability to use abstract terms. There is generally an impairment in the social use of both verbal and gestural language. Problems in social relationships are most severe before the age of five years and include an impairment in the development of eye-to-eye gaze, social attachments, and cooperative play. Ritualistic behaviour is usual and may include abnormal routines, resistance to change, attachment to odd objects and stereotyped patterns of play. The capacity for abstract or symbolic thought and for imaginative play is diminished. **Intelligence** ranges from severely subnormal to normal or above. Performance is usually better on tasks involving rote memory or visuospatial **skills** than on those requiring symbolic or linguistic skills [MDG]. The cause is probably a biologically based form of cognitive **defect** affecting the development of language. The prognosis is generally poor and related most closely to the level of intelligence.

Comment: This syndrome was reported originally by Kanner in 1943, who described most of the accepted features of the condition.

Synonyms: childhood autism; Kanner's syndrome; infantile psychosis (deprecated).

'bad trip' (ICD: 305.3) A colloquialism for an acute **panic** reaction occurring as an unwanted adverse effect of hallucinogenic drugs, usually characterized by fear of death and of insanity and by various other abnormal experiences, e.g., distortions of body image, or sensations of breathlessness or paralysis. The reaction is extremely unpleasant but usually short-lived and varies in intensity, occasionally leading to accidents and suicide attempts.

See also: hallucinogens abuse.

barbiturate and tranquillizer abuse (ICD: 305.4) Taking of such drugs to the detriment of one's health or social functioning, in doses above, or for periods beyond, those normally regarded as therapeutic [MDG].

bestiality (ICD: 302.1) Sexual intercourse with animals.

bipolar disorder (ICD: 296.2; 296.3) A form of phasic affective illness with both **manic** and **depressive** phenomena, in contrast to the **unipolar (monopolar)** form of affective illnesses. Since the introduction of the terms monopolar and bipolar by Leonhard in 1957, the clinical, genetic and biological features underlying this distinction have been regarded by many as justifying an independent status for each of the two syndromes, monopolar and bipolar disorder, replacing the term **manic-depressive psychosis**. This contention remains to be firmly established.

See also: manic-depressive psychosis, circular type but currently manic, and manic-depressive psychosis, manic type.

borderline state (ICD: 295.5) A poorly defined term employed with reference to three groups of mental aberration. These are (1) an incomplete form of **schizophrenia**, virtually synonymous with **schizoid personality disorder**; (2) a general category of personality or character disorder, construed in psychoanalytical terms as a disturbance of ego function; (3) a more specific form of **personality disorder** characterized by defective affectional relationships, a deficient self-identity, feelings of depressive loneliness and a tendency to outbursts of anger. None of these categories has been established as a valid clinical syndrome.

bouffée délirante (ICD: 298.3) A term used to designate acute psychotic episodes originally thought to occur in **psychopathic personalities** (dégénérés). The original description of the clinical picture contained five cardinal characteristics: abruptness of onset, a variety of fully formed **delusions** with occasional **hallucinosis**, some **clouding of consciousness** associated with emotional instability, an absence of physical signs, and a rapid complete remission. More recently, other features have been emphasized: the possibility of precipitation by psychosocial stressors; the high incidence or recurrence of episodes after asymptomatic intervals; the nosological independence of the episode from **schizophrenia**, though a chronic schizophrenic state may develop after one or more relapses.

Comment: The term was first introduced in 1886 by Legrain and adopted by Magnan.

See also: schizophrenic episode, acute; reactive psychosis; schizophreniform psychosis.

Briquet's disorder (ICD: 300.8) According to DSM-III[1], a syndrome characterized by polysymptomatology and frequent unnecessary medicosurgical contacts without evidence of organic disease, commencing before the age of 30 and thought to occur principally in genetically predisposed women of lower socioeconomic class. The nosological status of the syndrome and its relations to **hysteria** with **conversion** reaction, on the one hand, and to **hypochondriasis**, on the other, have still to be established.

Comment: The term is named (incorrectly) after Pierre Briquet (1796-1881), who wrote a classical monograph on hysteria in all its manifestations.

bulimia (ICD: 307.5) An irresistible urge to consume large quantities of food, occasionally attributable to an endocrine disturbance but most frequently associated with a functional eating disorder. Characteristically, the episode of 'binge eating' is followed by self-induced vomiting or purging, and by self-deprecation.

See also: anorexia nervosa.

cardiac neurosis (ICD: 306.2) (deprecated) A group of cardiovascular symptoms, frequently associated with dysfunctions in other physiological systems, presenting as autonomic manifestations of an **anxiety** state. Common complaints like palpitations, thoracic apical pain, breathlessness, dizzi-

---

[1] [DSM III] = *Diagnostic and statistical manual of mental disorders*, 3rd ed. Washington, DC, Ameri. can Psychiatric Association, 1980.

ness on postural change or effort, sweating and flushes, and fatigue, may mask the underlying anxiety and **panic** attacks.

Comment: The syndrome was first described during military campaigns in the 19th and early 20th centuries, and has been known under a variety of names, e.g., 'irritable heart' (Da Costa, 1871), 'effort syndrome' (Lewis, 1917), and 'neurocirculatory asthenia' (Oppenheimer, 1918).

Synonyms (deprecated): cardiovascular neurosis; Da Costa's syndrome; effort phobia; effort syndrome; irritable heart; neurocirculatory asthenia; soldier's heart.

catastrophic stress (ICD: 308) A reaction to exceptionally severe physical or mental **stress**, characterized by a breakdown of coping behaviour, intense **anxiety** and shock. The term has also been applied to the state of **agitation** and helplessness exhibited by patients with cerebral damage when confronted with tasks beyond their competence (Goldstein, 1878-1965).

See also: acute reactions to stress.

character neurosis (ICD: 301) (deprecated) A psychoanalytical concept derived from a typology constructed from the interpretation of character traits as either derivations of phases of development, or the analogues of particular symptoms. Thus the former would include the oral or anal character; the latter would include the hysterical or obsessional character. According to this concept, the manifestations of character neurosis are intermediate between normal character traits and neurotic symptoms (Jones, 1938).

See also: personality disorders.

childhood psychosis, atypical (ICD: 299.8) A variety of infantile psychotic disorders which may show some, but not all of the features of **infantile autism**. Symptoms may include **stereotyped repetitive movements**, **hyperkinesis**, self-injury, retarded speech development, **echolalia** and impaired social relationships. Such disorders may occur in children of any level of **intelligence** but are particularly common in those with **mental retardation** [MDG].

cognitive or personality change following organic brain damage, other than frontal lobe syndrome (ICD: 310.1) Chronic, mild states of memory disturbance and intellectual deterioration, often accompanied by increased **irritability**, querulousness, lassitude and complaints of physical weakness. These states are often associated with old age, and may precede more severe states due to brain damage classifiable under **dementia** of any type [MDG].

Synonyms: mild memory disturbance; organic psychosyndrome of non-psychotic severity.

compensation neurosis (ICD: 310.2) An ill-defined, heterogeneous assortment of neurotic symptoms with a marked somatic tint (**anxiety**, **irritability**, postural dizziness, headache, poor concentration, visual difficulties, sleep disturbances, sexual problems, intractable pain), all attributed by the patient to the effects of an accident or other injury (especially involving the head) and presented as a motive for litigation aimed at compensation. The condition, first described by Charcot (1873) and by Oppenheim (1889), has been claimed to occur more frequently in men, in the less educated and less skilled occupational groups, and in people with pre-existing emotional difficulties. Although the 'secondary gain' motive often features prominently as a unifying theme for the variable symptomatology, the psychological causation of the complaints may be overinterpreted and the possible contribution of organic factors overlooked. The nosological status of the condition remains, therefore, uncertain.
Synonyms: accident neurosis; litigation neurosis; traumatic neurosis; post-traumatic neurosis.

confusional state, acute (ICD: 293.0) Short-lived transient psychotic condition, lasting hours or days [MDG]. Unless specified as 'reactive' confusion, the term refers to **organic** states, e.g. **delirium** or **twilight** state.
Synonyms: acute psycho-organic syndrome; acute organic reaction (deprecated).

confusional state, subacute (ICD: 293.1) Transient organic psychotic condition in which the symptoms, usually less florid than the acute state, last for several weeks or longer, during which time they may show marked fluctuations in intensity [MDG].
Synonyms: amentia (deprecated); subacute delirium; subacute psycho-organic syndrome.

confusion, reactive (ICD: 298.2) Mental disorders with **clouded consciousness, disorientation** (though less marked than in organic confusion) and diminished accessibility often accompanied by excessive activity and apparently provoked by emotional **stress** [MDG].
Synonyms: psychogenic confusion; psychogenic twilight state.

conversion reaction (ICD: 300.1) The manifestation of an essentially psychological complex of ideas, wishes and feelings in terms of somatic (motor and/or sensory) dysfunction which represents an intrapsychic symbolic conflict or wish fulfilment. The phenomena are most characteristically features of hysterical states. In psychoanalytical theory it is the affect associated with a complex set of ideas that is converted into physical symptoms.

culture shock (ICD: 309.2) A state of social isolation, **anxiety** and **depression** resulting when a person is suddenly placed in an alien culture or re-enters his or her own culture after a prolonged absence, or has divided loyalties to two or more cultures. It is common among immigrants, but can occur also when life circumstances change radically within a society.

cyclothymia (ICD: 301.1) A term introduced by Kahlbaum to designate the milder forms of depressive and elated mood-swings conceived as phases of a single, **manic-depressive** disease. Its adjectival form, cyclothymic, is applied to **personality disorders** characterized by affective anomalies.
See also: affective personality disorder.
Synonym: manic-depressive illness.

delays in development, specific (ICD: 315) A group of disorders in which a specific delay in development is the main feature. In each case development is related to biological maturation but it is also influenced by nonbiological factors and the term carries no etiological implications.
Synonym: specific developmental disorders.

delinquency (ICD: 312.1, 312.3) A loose term applied technically to various forms of misbehaviour amounting to legal offences committed by children and young people. Among the important contributory factors are socioeconomic and familiar influences, group environment, and such personality characteristics as immaturity, egocentricity, and a poorly developed capacity to form personal relationships.
See also: delinquent act.

delirium (ICD: 291.0, 293.0) An etiologically nonspecific cerebral organic syndrome characterized by impaired **consciousness** with **disorientation**, morbid perceptual and affective phenomena, high arousal, and increased psychomotor activity. Illusions, **hallucinations**, **delusions**, and restlessness accompany cognitive impairment. The delirious state may be acute or subacute, and is usually of fluctuating intensity.
Synonyms: acute organic confusional state.

delirium tremens (ICD: 291.0) Acute or subacute organic psychotic states in **alcohol-dependent** people characterized by **clouded consciousness, disorientation**, fear, illusions, **delusions, hallucinations** of any kind, notably visual and tactile, and restlessness, tremor and sometimes fever [MDG].
Comment: The syndrome was first described in 1813 by Thomas Sutton (1767-1835).
Synonyms: alcoholic delirium; alcohol withdrawal delirium.

dementia (ICD: 290, 294) A syndrome, usually of a chronic or progressive nature, in which there is impairment of **orientation**, memory, **comprehension**, calculation, **learning capacity** and **judgement** and which is associated with an organic condition affecting cerebral function [MDG].

dementia, arteriosclerotic (ICD: 290.4) Dementia attributable, because of physical signs (on examination of the central nervous system) to degenerative arterial disease of the brain. Symptoms suggesting a focal lesion in the brain are common. There may be a fluctuating or patchy intellectual **defect** with insight, and an intermittent course is common. Clinical differentiation from **senile** or **presenile dementia**, with which it may coexist, may be very difficult or impossible [MDG].
Synonyms: multi-infarct dementia; vascular dementia.

dementia, presenile (ICD: 290.1) Dementia occurring usually before the age of 65 in patients with relatively rare forms of diffuse or lobar cerebral atrophy (Alzheimer's disease or Pick's disease of the brain) [MDG]. The clinical manifestations and course are as in **senile dementia**.
Synonyms: brain syndrome with presenile brain disease (deprecated); circumscribed atrophy of the brain (deprecated); primary degenerative dementia, presenile onset; presenile dementia, Alzheimer/Pick type.

dementia, senile, with acute confusional state (ICD: 290.3) Senile dementia with a superimposed reversible episode of **acute confusional state** [MDG].
Synonyms: primary degenerative dementia, senile onset, with delirium; senile dementia, Alzheimer type (with delirium).

dementia, senile, depressed or paranoid type (ICD: 290.2) A type of senile **dementia** characterized by development in advanced old age, progressive in nature, in which a variety of **delusions** and **hallucinations** of a persecutory, depressive and somatic content are also present. Disturbance of the sleep/waking cycle and preoccupation with dead people are often particularly prominent [MDG].
Synonyms: primary degenerative dementia, senile onset, with depression/ delusions; senile dementia, Alzheimer type, with depression/ delusions.

dementia, senile, simple type (ICD: 290.0) Dementia occurring usually after the age of 65 in which any cerebral pathology other than of senile atrophic change, **Alzheimer's disease** or other rare forms of cerebral atrophy, can be reasonably excluded [MDG]. The course is progressive, the average duration of the disease being about seven years, without remissions. Clinically, the initial stage typically presents with mnemic disturbances, spatial disorientation and either a pronounced lack of spontaneous activity or purposeless hyperactivity; the later stages witness the appearance of

hypertonic-atonic motor disturbances, and of focal symptoms, particularly agnosia, aphasia, logoclonia and apraxia, leading terminally to profound dementia.
Synonyms: primary degenerative dementia, senile onset, uncomplicated; senile dementia, Alzheimer type, simple.

depersonalization syndrome (ICD: 300.6) A rare neurotic disorder with an unpleasant state of disturbed perception in which parts of one's own body are experienced as changed in their quality, unreal, remote or automatized. Patients are aware of the subjective nature of the changes they experience. Depersonalization may occur as a feature of several mental disorders including **depression, obsessive-compulsive neurosis, anxiety** and **schizophrenia**.
Synonym: derealization (neurotic).

depression (ICD: 290.2, 293, 294.8, 295.7, 296, 298.0, 300, 301.1, 308.0, 309.0, 309.1, 311) In lay terminology, a state of gloom, despondency or sadness which may or may not denote ill-health. In a medical context the term refers to a morbid mental state dominated by a lowering of mood and often accompanied by a variety of associated symptoms, particularly **anxiety**, **agitation**, feelings of unworthiness, suicidal ideas, hypobulia, psychomotor retardation, and various somatic symptoms, physiological dysfunctions (e.g., insomnia), and complaints. Depression, as a symptom or a syndrome, is a major or significant feature in a variety of disease categories. The term is widely and sometimes imprecisely used to designate a symptom, a syndrome, and a disease state.
Synonym: melancholia (deprecated).

depression, neurotic (ICD: 300.4) A **neurotic disorder** characterized by disproportionate **depression** which has usually recognizably followed a distressing experience; it does not include among its features **delusions** or **hallucinations**, and there is often preoccupation with the psychic trauma which preceded the illness, e.g., loss of a cherished person or possession. **Anxiety** is also frequently present and mixed states of anxiety and depression should be included here. The distinction between depressive neurosis and psychosis should be made not only upon the degree of depression but also on the presence or absence of other neurotic and psychotic characteristics and upon the degree of disturbance of the patient's behaviour.
Synonyms: depressive reaction (deprecated); neurotic depressive state; depression, reactive (deprecated).

depression, unipolar (monopolar) (ICD: 296.1) A form of recurrent depressive illness without evidence of manic features. Absence of family history of **mania** in first degree relatives, as well as characteristic biological and therapeutic responses have been suggested as confirmatory evidence. The

independence of this pattern of disorder from **bipolar affective disorder (manic-depressive illness)** is not firmly established.
Synonyms: periodic depression; recurrent depression.

depressive disorder (ICD: 311) A state of **depression**, usually of moderate but occasionally of marked intensity, which has no specifically **manic-depressive** or other psychotic depressive features and which does not appear to be associated with stressful events or other features specified under **neurotic depression**.
Synonyms: depressive illness; depressive state.

depressive reaction, brief (ICD: 309.0) State of **depression**, not specifiable as manic-depressive, psychotic or neurotic, generally transient, in which the depressive symptoms are usually closely related in time and content to some stressful event [MDG].

depressive reaction, prolonged (ICD: 309.1) States of **depression**, not specifiable as **manic-depressive**, psychotic or neurotic, generally long-lasting; usually developing in association with prolonged exposure to a **stressful** situation [MDG].

developmental disorder, mixed (ICD: 315.5) A delay in the development of one specific skill (e.g., reading, arithmetic, speech or coordination) associated with lesser delays in other skills. The mixed category should be used only where the mixture of delayed skill is such that no one skill is predominantly affected [MDG].

developmental speech or language disorder (ICD: 315.3) Disorders in which the main feature is a serious impairment in the development of speech or language (syntax or semantics) which is not explicable in terms of general intellectual retardation. Most commonly there is a delay in the development of normal word-sound production resulting in defects of articulation. Omissions or substitutions of consonants are most frequent. There may also be a delay in the production of spoken language. Rarely, there is also a developmental delay in the comprehension of sounds. Includes cases in which delay is largely due to environmental privation [MDG].
Synonyms: developmental aphasia; dyslalia; developmental language disorder, expressive/receptive type.

disintegrative psychosis (ICD: 299.1) A heterogeneous group of conditions usually commencing at the age of three or four years when, after general premonitory symptoms, the hitherto normal child develops, over a few months, loss of speech and of social skills accompanied by hyperactivity, **stereotyped motor behaviour**, a severe impairment of emotional response, and, usually but not necessarily, of intellectual capacity. Clinical evidence of neurological disease is uncommon but the psychosis may result from a variety

of illnesses which damage the brain (e.g., measles encephalitis). The outcome is poor, most children becoming mentally retarded and incapable of speech.
Comment: The syndrome was originally described as 'dementia infantilis' by Heller in 1930.
Synonyms: Heller's syndrome; childhood onset pervasive developmental disorder.

dissociative reaction or state (ICD: 300.1) A condition resulting from the coexistence of conscious and unconscious mental processes which are split or poorly integrated, resulting in inconsistencies of thought or conduct. As a 'mental mechanism', dissociation may account for the psychological phenomena associated with several conditions, including **hysteria**, some forms of **schizophrenia**, hypnosis, **sleep-walking**, **fugue** and some epileptic phenomena.
See also: hysteria; multiple personality; sleep-walking; narrowing of the field of consciousness.

disturbance of conduct and emotions, mixed (ICD: 312.3) Disorders involving behaviours listed for **disturbances of conduct, unsocialized and socialized**, but in which there is also considerable emotional disturbance as shown for example by **anxiety**, misery or **obsessive** manifestations [MDG].
Synonym: neurotic delinquency.

disturbances of conduct (ICD: 312) Disorders mainly involving **aggressiveness** and destructive behaviour, and disorders involving **deliquency**. The term should be used for abnormal behaviour, in individuals of any age, which gives rise to social disapproval but which is not part of any other psychiatric condition. Minor emotional disturbances may also be present. To be included, the behaviour (as judged by its frequency, severity, and type of associations with other symptoms) must be abnormal in its context. Disturbances of conduct are distinguished from an **adjustment reaction** by a longer duration and by a lack of close relationship in time and content to **stress**. They differ from a **personality disorder** by the absence of deeply ingrained maladaptive patterns of behaviour present from adolescence or earlier [MDG].
Synonym: conduct disorders.

disturbance of conduct, compulsive (ICD: 312.2) Disorder of conduct or delinquent act which is specifically compulsive in origin.
Synonym: conduct disorder, compulsive.

disturbance of conduct, socialized (ICD: 312.1) Disorders in individuals who have acquired the values or behaviour of a delinquent peer group to whom they are loyal and with whom they characteristically steal, play truant, or stay out late at night. There may also be promiscuity [MDG].
Synonym: group delinquency.

disturbance of conduct, unsocialized (ICD: 312.0) Disorders character-ized by behaviours such as defiance, disobedience, quarrelsomeness, **ag-gression**, destructive behaviour, tantrums, solitary stealing, lying, teasing, bullying, and disturbed relationships with others. The defiance may some-times take the form of sexual misconduct [MDG].
Synonyms: conduct disorder, undersocialized, aggressive/nonaggressive; unsocialized aggressive disorder.

disturbance of emotions specific to childhood and adolescence (ICD: 313) Less well-differentiated emotional disorders characteristic of the childhood period. Where the emotional disorder takes the form of a **neurotic disorder**, the appropriate ICD coding (300) should be made. This category differs from the category **acute reactions to stress** in terms of longer duration, and by the lack of close relationship in time and content to stress [MDG].

disturbance of emotions specific to childhood and adolescence, with anxiety and fearfulness (ICD: 313.0) Ill-defined emotional disorders characteristic of childhood in which the main symptoms involve **anxiety** and fearfulness. Many cases of school refusal or **elective mutism** might be included here [MDG].
Synonym: overanxious reaction of childhood or adolescence.

disturbance of emotions specific to childhood and adolescence, with misery and unhappiness (ICD: 313.1) Emotional disorders charac-teristic of childhood in which the main symptoms involve misery and unhappiness. There may also be eating and sleep disturbances [MDG].

disturbance of emotions specific to childhood and adolescence, with sensitivity, shyness and social withdrawal (ICD: 313.2) Emotional disorders characteristic of childhood in which the main symptoms involve sensitivity, shyness, or **social withdrawal**. Some cases of **elective mutism** might be included here [MDG].
Synonym: withdrawing reaction in childhood or adolescence.

Down's syndrome (ICD: 758.0) An abnormality of an autosomal chromo-some, associated with **mental retardation** and characteristic physical features. In most cases the anomaly consists in trisomy of a chromosome of the G group; the remainder may exhibit D/G translocation, G/G translocation or mosaicism. The incidence of Down's syndrome has been estimated as close to 1 in 550 live births, with a relationship to late maternal age. The degree of mental retardation varies, but the IQ level on standard tests is rarely above 70. Physical features include characteristic 'mongoloid' facies, single palmar creases, a large fissured tongue, hypotonia, retarded growth and congenital cardiac and gastrointestinal defects. The condition was originally described by John Langdon Haydon Down (1828-1896).

Synonyms: Mongolism (deprecated); Langdon Down's disease (deprecated); autosomal trisomy G; congenital acromicria (deprecated); trisomy 21.

drug abuse (ICD: 305) The self-administration of a medicinal or pleasurable substance in a quantity or manner that impairs health or social functioning. The term has pejorative overtones so it is advisable to restrict its use to indicate the malevolence of an individual, or of his or her behaviour. See also: hallucinogens abuse.

drug abuse, nondependent (ICD: 305) Self-administration of a drug without dependence (as defined in 'drug dependence' below), to the detriment of one's health or social functioning. Drug abuse may be secondary to a psychiatric disorder [MDG]. The term, and the concept on which it is based, have been contested in the light of evidence that dependent and nondependent abuse of drugs cannot be reliably distinguished.

drug dependence (ICD: 304) A state, psychic and sometimes also physical, resulting from taking a drug, characterized by behavioural and other responses that always include a **compulsion** to take a drug on a continuous or periodic basis in order to experience its psychic effects, and sometimes to avoid the discomfort of its absence. Tolerance may or may not be present. A person may be dependent on more than one drug [MDG].
Synonyms: drug addiction; toxicomania (deprecated).

drug-induced paranoid and/or hallucinatory states (ICD: 292.1) States of more than a few days' but not usually of more than a few months', duration, associated with large or prolonged intake of drugs, notably of the amphetamine and LSD groups. Auditory **hallucinations** usually predominate, and there may be **anxiety** and restlessness [MDG].

drug intoxication, pathological (ICD: 292.2) Individual idiosyncratic reactions to comparatively small quantities of drugs, other than hallucinogens, which take the form of acute, brief psychotic states of any type [MDG].

drug psychoses (ICD: 292) Syndromes of either predominantly **organic** or predominantly nonorganic type, which are due to consumption of drugs (notably amphetamines, barbiturates, and the opiate and LSD groups) and solvents. Some of the syndromes in this ICD-9 group are not as severe as most conditions labelled 'psychotic' but they are included for practical reasons [MDG].
Synonyms: toxic psychoses due to use of drugs; pharmacogenic psychoses.

drug withdrawal syndrome (ICD: 292.0) State associated with the discontinuation of the taking of a drug, ranging from severe, as specified for alcohol **(delirium tremens)**, to less severe states characterized by one or more symptoms such as convulsions, tremor, **anxiety**, restlessness, gastrointestinal and muscular complaints, and mild **disorientation** and memory disturbance. Synonym: abstinence syndrome.

drunkenness, pathological (ICD: 291.4) Acute psychotic episodes induced by relatively small amounts of alcohol. These are regarded as individual idiosyncratic reactions to alcohol, not due to excessive consumption, and without conspicuous neurological signs of intoxication [MDG]. Synonym: alcohol idiosyncratic intoxication.

dyslexia, developmental (ICD: 315.0) A disorder manifested by difficulty in reading and spelling, despite adequate **intelligence**, conventional instruction, and sociocultural opportunity. It is attributable to a constitutional cognitive disability.
See also: reading retardation, specific.

dyspareunia, psychogenic (ICD: 302.7) Genital pain during the act of sexual intercourse, usually in women, with no apparent physical cause.

elective mutism (ICD: 309.8) A condition exhibited by children who, although being able to talk and comprehend language, remain silent in the presence of particular individuals and in certain environments, usually related to school. In most cases any associated abnormalities are in the spheres of temperament and emotion, but some of the children also suffer from minor disorders of speech, language, or both.
Comment: The term was introduced by Tramer in 1934.

encopresis (ICD: 307.7) A disorder, most common in children, in which the main manifestation is the persistent voluntary or involuntary passage of formed faeces of normal or near-normal consistency, into places not intended for that purpose, in the individual's own sociocultural setting. Sometimes the child has failed to gain bowel control, and sometimes the child has gained control but becomes encopretic again later. There may be a variety of associated psychiatric symptoms, and there may be smearing of faeces. The condition would not usually be diagnosed under the age of four years [MDG].

enuresis (ICD: 307.6) A disorder, most common in children, in which the main manifestation is a persistent involuntary voiding of urine by day or night which is considered abnormal for the age of the individual. Sometimes the child will have failed to gain bladder control and in other cases he or she will have gained control and then lost it. Episodic or fluctuating enuresis should be included. The disorder would not usually be diagnosed under the age of four years [MDG].

epileptic dementia (ICD: 294.1) (deprecated) An incorrect term formerly used to describe any state of **dementia** secondary to the repetition of epileptic

seizures. Since the dementia is not due to recurring epileptic seizures but rather to an associated progressive encephalopathy, the term should be replaced by 'dementia in epilepsy' [DE].
Synonym: epileptic insanity (deprecated).

epileptic psychosis, acute (ICD: 294.8) (deprecated) A term describing the acute psychotic manifestations, usually lasting from several days to a few weeks, that are liable to occur in an epileptic independently of seizures and of ictal or postictal **confusional states**. These manifestations, which usually take the form of an **acute paranoid reaction**, are encountered mostly in people with seizures of temporal-lobe origin, usually during spontaneous periods of remission or remissions produced by anticonvulsive treatment. They are often accompanied by the disappearance of interictal electroencephalogram (EEG) discharges ('forced normalization'). The fact that such manifestations are not necessarily related to seizures, and occur in only some epileptics, indicates that the strict relation suggested by the term 'acute epileptic psychosis' cannot be demonstrated. Preference should therefore, be given to the expression 'acute psychotic episode in an epileptic' or 'acute psychosis in an epileptic'.

Comment: In ICD-9, 'epileptic psychosis NOS' is listed as an inclusion term under 294.8 (other states that fulfil the criteria of an **organic** psychosis but do not take the form of a confusional state, a nonalcoholic **Korsakov's psychosis** or a **dementia**). This provision does not allow a distinction between acute and chronic forms [DE].

epileptic psychosis, chronic (ICD: 294.8) Chronic hallucinatory **paranoid** psychosis occurring in subjects with epilepsy, particularly temporal-lobe epilepsy. It is often characterized by religious or mystical **delusions** and tends to occur in subjects whose seizures are tapering off, whether spontaneously or in response to treatment. Chronic epileptic psychosis is rare and it is difficult to distinguish from the 'functional' paranoid psychoses, although in the epileptic variety affect and social integration are sometimes well-preserved.

The relationship between epilepsy and chronic psychosis is neither simple nor clear. On the one hand, the psychotic phenomena are directly related to epilepsy of the temporal lobe, probably of the dominant hemisphere; occur in inverse proportion to the presence and frequency of temporal lobe seizures; and are independent of the presence of associated brain lesions.

This is all evidence in favour of the epileptic nature of the psychotic manifestations. On the other hand, it would be more appropriate to use the expression 'chronic psychosis in an epileptic individual', since numerous factors — organic, psychological (the reliving of previous experiences during some seizures), sociological (rejection by society, low status of the epileptic), and pharmacological (long-term anti-convulsant therapy, which disturbs

folic acid metabolism) — may play a part in the causation of the psychoses observed in epileptics [DE].
See also: 'Comment' under 'epileptic psychosis, acute'.

epileptic twilight state (ICD: 293.0) A transient psychic change occurring during or after an epileptic seizure, usually one of temporal lobe origin, and characterized by reduced alertness with **narrowing of the field of consciousness** resulting in a 'hazy' and 'blurred' perception of the surroundings. Such states may be classed as intermediate between confusional states, in which dissolution of consciousness is more complete, and dreamy states, in which fantasy is prevalent [DE].
See also: confusion; dream-like states.

feminism in boys (ICD: 302.6) Adoption by preadolescent boys of appearance, clothes and behaviour typical of the female sex. Early effeminate behaviour in boys can be a precursor or predictor of adult homosexuality.

fetishism (ICD: 302.8) A condition in which erotic arousal is related to inanimate objects such as clothes, shoes, articles of adornment, or parts of the body (e.g., hair, feet) in preference to, or as a substitute for, sexual intercourse.

frontal lobe syndrome (ICD: 310.0) Changes in behaviour following damage to the frontal areas of the brain or following interference with the connections of those areas. There is generally diminution of self-control, foresight, creativity and spontaneity, which may be manifest as increased **irritability**, selfishness and lack of concern for others. Conscientiousness and powers of concentration are often diminished, but measurable deterioration of intellect or memory is not necessarily present. The overall picture is often one of emotional dullness, lack of drive and slowness. Particularly in people with previously energetic, restless or aggressive characteristics, there may be a change towards **impulsiveness**, boastfulness, temper outbursts, silly fatuous humour, and the development of unrealistic ambitions; the direction of change usually depends upon the previous personality. A considerable degree of recovery is possible and may continue over the course of several years [MDG].
Synonyms: lobotomy syndrome (deprecated); postleucotomy syndrome (deprecated).

Ganser's syndrome (ICD: 300.1) A form of pseudodementia with a core symptom of 'approximate answers' or 'talking past the point' (Vorbeireden, réponse à côté). Associated features include fluctuating disturbances of **consciousness**, **hallucinosis**, and memory **defects**. The syndrome was originally (1898) regarded as a manifestation of **hysteria** in some cases, especially those with forensic overtones; it may be precipitated by emotional disturbance and

be accompanied by hysterical stigmata, resolving abruptly with subsequent **amnesia** for the episode. However, both the functional psychoses and organic cerebral disease can be associated with Ganser's syndrome, which in fact is found more frequently in mental hospitals than in prisons.
See also: hysterical psychosis.

gender role disorder (ICD: 302.6) A condition in which conflict, with resulting distress, is experienced between the external appearance and orientation of assigned sex on the one hand, and biological sex and/or gender identity on the other. Cultural factors may be prepotent. Trans-sexualism exemplifies the condition.

general paralysis of the insane (ICD: 294.1) A form of tertiary neurosyphilis in which neurological (oculomotor paresis, Argyll Robertson pupil, optic atrophy, tremor, ataxia, dysarthria, loss of bladder and bowel control) and psychopathological (**dementia**, expansive, paranoid or depressive **delusions**, deterioration of social behaviour) syndromes arise on the basis of a progressive infiltrative polioencephalitis leading to atrophy, which is caused by the direct invasion of the brain parenchyma by the spirochaete. If untreated, the course of the disease is progressive, resulting in severe dementia and, ultimately, death.
Comments: From a peak in the early and mid-19th century, the incidence of the disease has shown a dramatic decline over the last few decades. The condition was described by Bayle (1822) but the term was introduced by Delaye (1824).
Synonyms: general paresis; dementia paralytica; paralysis progressiva; Bayle's disease.

Gilles de la Tourette syndrome (ICD: 307.2) A rare disorder occurring in individuals of any level of intelligence in which facial **tics** and tic-like throat noises become more marked and more generalized and in which, later, whole words or short sentences (often with an obscene content) are ejaculated spasmodically and involuntarily. There is some overlap with other varieties of tic [MDG].
Synonym: Tourette's syndrome.

grief reaction (ICD: 309.0) A response by a bereaved person to the loss, that characteristically proceeds from a phase of shock and bewilderment, via a depressive preoccupation with the deceased, to a gradual period of resolution. Deviations from this sequence are common and morbid patterns of grieving may constitute a frank depressive illness.
Synonyms: bereavement reaction; brief depressive reaction related to bereavement; uncomplicated bereavement.

hallucinogens abuse (ICD: 305.3) Acute, self-induced hallucinogen intoxication motivated by a desire to experience the consciousness and perception-altering effects of the drug.
See also: drug abuse.
Synonym: LSD (or other hallucinogen) reaction.

hallucinosis (ICD: 291.3) A relatively rare, acute or chronic, state in which recurrent or persistent **hallucinations** in clear **consciousness** constitute the dominant clinical feature. It is attributable principally to misuse of alcohol or other centrally acting drugs but may occur, less commonly, in association with forms of cerebral disorder, and in the functional psychoses.
Synonym: hallucinatory state.

hospitalism in children (ICD: 309.8) A syndrome closely related to anaclitic **depression,** developing in infants in hospital who are separated from their mothers or mother-surrogates for long periods of time. It is characterized by listlessness, unresponsiveness, emaciation and pallor, poor appetite and disturbed sleep, febrile episodes, lack of sucking habits, and an appearance of unhappiness. The disorder is reversible if the mother, or mother-surrogate, and child are reunited within 2−3 weeks.
Synonym: reactive attachment disorder of infancy.

hyperkinesis with developmental delay (ICD: 314.1) Cases in which the hyperkinetic **syndrome of childhood** (see below) is associated with speech delay, clumsiness, reading difficulties, or other delays in specific skills.
Synonyms: attention deficit disorder with hyperactivity, associated with developmental disorder; developmental disorder of hyperkinesis.

hyperkinetic conduct disorder (ICD: 314.2) Cases in which the hyperkinetic syndrome of childhood (see below) is associated with marked **conduct** disturbance but not **developmental delay** [MDG].
Synonym: attention deficit disorder with hyperactivity, associated with conduct disorder.

hyperkinetic syndrome of childhood (ICD: 314) Disorders in which the essential features are short attention-span and distractibility. In early childhood the most striking symptom is disinhibited, poorly organized and poorly regulated extreme overactivity, but in adolescence this may be replaced by underactivity. **Impulsiveness**, marked **mood** fluctuations and **aggressiveness** are also common symptoms. Delays in the development of specific **skills** are often present and disturbed, poor relationships are common [MDG].
Synonym: attention deficit disorder with hyperactivity.

hypochondriasis (ICD: 300.7) A **neurotic disorder** in which the conspicuous features are excessive concern with one's health in general, or the integrity and functioning of some part of one's body, or, less frequently, one's mind. It is usually associated with **anxiety** and depression. It may occur as a feature of severe mental disorder and in that case should be classified in the corresponding major category [MDG].

hysteria (ICD: 300.1) A mental disorder in which motives, of which the patient seems unaware, produce either a **restriction of the field of consciousness** or disturbances of motor or sensory function which may seem to have psychological advantage or symbolic value. It may be characterized by **conversion** phenomena or **dissociative** phenomena. In the conversion form the chief or only symptoms consist of **psychogenic** disturbance of function in some part of the body, e.g., paralysis, tremor, blindness, deafness or seizures. In the dissociative variety the most prominent feature is a narrowing of the field of consciousness which seems to serve an unconscious purpose and is commonly accompanied or followed by a selective **amnesia**. There may be dramatic but essentially superficial changes of **personality** sometimes taking the form of a **fugue**. Behaviour may mimic **psychosis** or, rather, the patient's idea of psychosis [MDG].
Synonyms: hysterical neurosis; conversion hysteria.

hysterical psychosis (ICD: 298.8) A term applied to a psychotic **reaction** to stressful circumstances occurring predominantly, but not exclusively, in individuals with hysterical personality traits. The illness is usually short-lived and may take one of several forms: **stupor**, **twilight** states, pseudodementia, **Ganser's syndrome**, **fugues**, and a **schizophrenia**-like state. Some culture-bound psychiatric syndromes e.g., latah, also have marked hysterical features.

idiocy (ICD: 318.2) (deprecated) A term employed widely but imprecisely from the 18th century onwards to designate conditions in which a primary weakness of the intellect exists from birth or early infancy, leading to a failure in educational attainment corresponding to age and social position. More recently the term has been applied more restrictively, to states of profound mental retardation.

imbecile (ICD: 318.0) (deprecated) A term characterizing a mentally subnormal individual with a level of intelligence intermediate between states of severe and moderate **mental retardation**.
See also: mental retardation, moderate.

induced psychosis (ICD: 297.3) Mainly delusional psychosis, usually chronic and often without florid features, which appears to have developed as a result of a close, if not dependent, relationship with another person who already has an established similar psychosis. The mental illness of the dominant member is most commonly paranoid. The morbid beliefs are induced in the other person and given up when the pair are separated. The **delusions** are at least partly shared [MDG]. Occasionally, several people are affected.

Synonyms: folie à deux; folie communiquée; folie imposée; folie induite; induced paranoid disorder; psychosis of association (deprecated); symbiontische Psychose.

insomnia of nonorganic origin (ICD: 307.4) Disorders of initiating or maintaining sleep, not associated with somatic disorders or dysfunctions and most commonly attributable to **anxiety**, tension, **affective** psychoses or adverse environmental factors.

Korsakov's psychosis, alcoholic (ICD: 291.1) A syndrome of prominent and lasting **reduction of memory span**, including striking loss of recent memory, disordered time appreciation and **confabulation**, occurring in alcohol-dependent people as a sequel to an acute alcoholic psychosis (especially **delirium tremens**), or more rarely, in the course of the **alcohol dependence syndrome**. It is usually accompanied by peripheral neuritis and may be associated with **Wernicke** encephalopathy [MDG].

Comment: First described in 1889 by Korsakov (1854-1900).

Synonyms: alcoholic polyneuritic psychosis; Korsakov's disease; alcoholic amnestic syndrome; Wernicke-Korsakov's syndrome.

Korsakov's psychosis or syndrome, nonalcoholic (ICD: 294.0) Symptoms described under 'Korsakov's psychosis, alcoholic' but not due to alcohol [MDG].

Synonyms: amnestic confabulary syndrome; dysmnesic syndrome.

learning difficulties, specific, other than reading and arithmetic retardation (ICD: 315.2) Disorders in which the main feature is a serious impairment in the development of **learning skills**, other than reading and arithmetic, which are not explicable in terms of general **mental retardation** or of inadequate schooling [MDG].

mania, unipolar (monopolar) (ICD: 296.0) A relatively rare condition of recurrent attacks of manic illness without depressive episodes.

Synonyms: periodic mania; hypomania.

manic-depressive psychosis, circular type but currently manic (ICD: 296.2, 296.3, 296.5) An **affective psychosis** which has appeared in both the depressive and the manic form, either alternating or separated by an interval of normality. The manic phase is far less frequent than the depressive phase [MDG].

Synonym: Bipolar disorder.

manic-depressive psychosis, circular type, mixed (ICD: 296.4) An **affective psychosis** in which both manic and depressive symptoms are present at the same time [MDG].
Synonym: mixed affective state.

manic-depressive psychosis, depressed type (ICD: 296.1) An **affective psychosis** in which there is a mood of gloom and wretchedness with some degree of **anxiety**. There is often reduced activity but there may be restlessness and **agitation**. There is a marked tendency to recurrence; in a few cases this may be at regular intervals [MDG].
Synonyms: depressive psychosis; endogenous depression; manic-depressive reaction, depressed; monopolar (unipolar) depression; psychotic depression.

manic-depressive psychosis, manic type (ICD: 296.0) Mental disorder characterized by states of **elation** or excitement out of keeping with the patient's circumstances and varying from enhanced liveliness (hypomania) to violent, almost uncontrollable excitement. **Aggression** and anger, **flight of ideas,** distractibility, impaired **judgement,** and **grandiose ideas** are common [MDG].
Synonyms: bipolar disorder, manic; mania; hypomania; manic episode; manic disorder; manic psychosis; hypomanic psychosis; manic-depressive psychosis or reaction; hypomanic; manic.

masochism (ICD: 302.8) A form of deviant sexual behaviour in which erotic pleasure is associated with the experience of pain, ill-treatment or humiliation. The term is also used more loosely to designate a **personality** type tending to self-induced suffering, discomfort or humiliation. Psychoanalytical theory distinguishes between erotogenic, feminine, and moral types of masochism.
Comment: The term refers to the Austrian writer Leopold von Sacher Masoch (1836-1895) whose novels contain descriptions of such behaviour.
See also: sadism.

melancholia (ICD: 296.1, 296.9) (deprecated) A term originating in the Hippocratic tradition (4th century BC) which was used to denote generally the depressive syndrome until the end of the 19th century. While Kraepelin and others restricted its use to refer only to depression in the elderly, Freud redefined it as a morbid counterpart of normal mourning. Amidst a general decline in its use, DSM-III resurrected the term by giving it yet another meaning in which the 'distinct quality of depressed mood' and precisely the contrast to normal mourning, are the prominent features. In view of this lack of precision, and the contradictory connotations, the continued use of the term is not recommended.

melancholia, involutional (ICD: 296.1) Depressive psychosis appearing during the involutional period (40-55 years for women, 50-65 years for men), in an individual with no history of previous **affective** illness. Although some symptoms and signs (such as delusions of guilt, sin or impoverishment, persecutory delusions, and **agitation** have been claimed to give involutional melancholia a distinctive clinical mark, epidemiological and family studies have failed to support its independent classification and have demonstrated its identity with **manic-depressive psychosis.**

mental retardation (general) (ICD: 317-319) A condition of arrested or incomplete development of the mind which is especially characterized by subnormality of **intelligence.** The assessment of intellectual level should be based on whatever information is available, including clinical evidence, adaptive behaviour and psychometric findings. Mental retardation often involves psychiatric disturbances and may often develop as a result of some physical disease or injury.
Synonyms: amentia (deprecated); mental deficiency; mental subnormality; oligophrenia.

mental retardation, mild (ICD: 317) Mental retardation corresponding to an IQ level of 50 to 70. Individuals with this level of subnormality are educable and usually acquire sufficient instrumental and social skills to enable them to adjust to the demands of daily life with minimum impairment.
Synonyms: feeble-minded (deprecated); high-grade defect (deprecated); mild mental subnormality; moron (deprecated); debility (deprecated).

mental retardation, moderate (ICD: 318.0) Mental retardation corresponding to an IQ level of 35 to 49. Individuals with this level of retardation usually acquire basic speech and can be trained for elementary self-care and simple occupational tasks, under supervision and guidance.
Synonym: imbecility (deprecated).

mental retardation, profound (ICD: 318.2) Mental retardation corresponding to an IQ level of below 20. Severe sensory—motor impairments are usually present, and acquisition of speech is not possible. In daily living such individuals require constant aid and supervision.
Synonym: idiocy (deprecated).

mental retardation, severe (ICD: 318.1) Mental retardation corresponding to an IQ level of 20 to 34. Individuals with this level of retardation usually suffer from impairment of motor and sensory development, and only acquire the rudiments of speech. Training in elementary self-care may be possible, though difficult, and constant close supervision of daily living is required.

moron (ICD: 317) (deprecated) A term used in North America to designate feeble-minded adults with a mental age of between 84 and 143 months or an IQ of between 50 and 74.

Comment: In other countries and languages the corresponding terms are derivations of the Latin debilitas.

motor retardation, specific (ICD: 315.4) Disorders in which the main feature is a serious impairment in the development of motor coordination which is not explicable in terms of general **mental retardation**. The clumsiness is commonly associated with perceptual difficulties [MDG].

Synonyms: clumsiness syndrome; dyspraxia syndrome.

neurasthenia (ICD: 300.5) A **neurotic disorder** characterized by fatigue, **irritability**, headache, **depression, insomnia**, difficulty in concentration, and lack of capacity for enjoyment (**anhedonia**). It may follow or accompany an infection or exhaustion, or arise from continued emotional **stress** [MDG].

Synonym: nervous debility (deprecated).

neurotic disorders (ICD: 300) The distinction between neurosis and **psychosis** is difficult and remains the subject of debate. However, it has been retained in ICD-9 in view of its wide use. Neurotic disorders are mental disorders, without any demonstrable organic basis in which the patient may have considerable **insight** and has unimpaired reality testing, in that he or she usually does not confuse his or her morbid subjective experiences and fantasies with external reality. Behaviour may be greatly affected although usually remaining within socially acceptable limits. **Personality** is not disorganized. The principal manifestations include excessive **anxiety, hysterical** symptoms, **phobias, obsessive** and **compulsive** symptoms, and **depression**.

Synonyms: neuroses; psychoneuroses (deprecated).

obsessive-compulsive disorder (ICD: 300.3) State in which the outstanding symptom is a feeling of subjective **compulsion** – which must be resisted – to carry out some action, to dwell on an idea, to recall an experience, or to ruminate on an abstract topic. Unwanted thoughts which intrude, the insistency of words or ideas, ruminations or trains of thought are perceived by the patient to be inappropriate or nonsensical. The obsessional urge or idea is recognized as alien to the **personality** but as coming from within the self. **Obsessional actions** may be quasi-ritual performances designed to relieve anxiety e.g., washing the hands to cope with contamination. Attempts to dispel the unwelcome thoughts or urges may lead to severe inner struggle, with intense anxiety [MDG].

Synonyms: anankastic neurosis; compulsive neurosis.

occupational neurosis (ICD: 300.8) (deprecated) A selective inhibition of the performance of specific, usually highly skilled actions, motor or mental, that are essential to a subject's occupation, in the absence of organic pathology. Examples are **writer's cramp**, musician's cramp, or accountant's sudden difficulty with mental arithmetic. Such dysfunction is usually a manifestation of an underlying **anxiety** state, and the term, with its implication of an independent status for the disorder, should be avoided.

oneirophrenia (ICD: 295.4) A syndrome described as occurring in acute **schizophrenic** illnesses, with some **clouding of consciousness** and a dream-like (oneiroid) state with vivid scenic **hallucinosis, catatonic** features and diminished contact with the real world.
Comment: The claim for an independent status of this syndrome has not
        found general support. The term was first introduced by Mayer-
        Gross in 1924 (as 'oneiroid state') and then used in 1945 by
        Meduna and McCulloch.
See also: dream-like state.

organic psychosyndrome, focal (partial) (ICD: 310.8) Any form of nonpsychotic mental disorder associated with localized damage to brain tissue.

paedophilia (ICD: 302.2) **Sexual deviation** in which an adult engages in sexual activity with a child of the same or opposite sex.
Synonym: paederosis.

panic disorder (ICD: 300.0) A term which is usually synonymous with **panic attack** but which may take such specific and unrelated forms as 'homosexual panic' and 'angor animi'. In DSM-III 'panic disorder' is a separate diagnostic entity within the group of 'anxiety states'.
Synonym: episodic paroxysmal anxiety.
See also: panic attack; panic state.

panic state (ICD: 300.0, 308.0) A sustained condition of overwhelming morbid **anxiety** affecting either an individual or a group to which the panic has been transmitted.
See also: panic disorder.

paranoia (ICD: 297.1) A rare chronic **psychosis** in which logically constructed systematized **delusions** have developed gradually without concomitant **hallucinations** or the **schizophrenic** type of disordered thinking. The delusions are mostly of grandeur (the paranoiac prophet or inventor), persecution or somatic abnormality [MDG].

paranoia querulans (ICD: 297.8) A state characterized by a quarrelsome **irritability** associated with a conviction of injustice and persecution, sometimes of **delusional** intensity, arising from real or imaginary wrongs, insults or injuries, and often leading to incessant litigation.
Synonym: litigious paranoia.

paranoid psychosis, psychogenic (ICD: 298.4) Psychogenic or reactive paranoid psychosis of any type which is more protracted than the acute reactions [MDG].
Synonym: protracted reactive paranoid psychosis.

paranoid reaction, acute (ICD: 298.3) Paranoid states apparently provoked by emotional **stress**. The stress is often misconstrued as an attack or threat. Such states are particularly prone to occur in prisoners or as acute reactions to a strange and threatening environment, e.g., in immigrants [MDG].

paranoid state, simple (ICD: 297.0) A psychosis, acute or chronic, not classifiable as **schizophrenia** or **affective psychosis**, in which **delusions**, especially of being influenced, persecuted or treated in some special way, are the main symptoms. The delusions are of a fairly fixed, elaborate and **systematized** kind [MDG].

paraphrenia (ICD: 297.2) (deprecated) In ICD-9, **paranoid psychosis** in which there are conspicuous **hallucinations**, often in several modalities. Affective symptoms and disordered thinking, if present, do not dominate the clinical picture and the **personality** is well preserved. In the early 19th century, Guislain used the term synonymously with 'folly' to denote delusional and hallucinatory states, but towards the end of the century Kraepelin designated it as a group of conditions intermediate between **paranoia** and paranoid **schizophrenia**. Qualifiers like 'involutional' or 'late' paraphrenia have added further dimensions to an already overexpanded concept. Because of its lack of specificity and precision, the use of this term should be discouraged.

personality, dependent (ICD: 301.6) A **personality disorder**, with or without asthenic features, with a low degree of self-esteem, a persistent tendency to avoid the assumption of responsibility, and an inclination to subordinate personal drives to those of other people.
See also: asthenic personality disorder.

personality, disinhibited ('haltlose') type (ICD: 301.8) A **personality disorder** characterized by lack of inhibition and control over urges, desires and impulses, especially manifest in the moral sphere: 'haltlose' (German) — lacking inhibition.

personality, eccentric (ICD: 301.8) A **personality disorder** characterized by an overvalued private system of beliefs or habits which are exaggerated in nature, sometimes fantastic, and held with fanatical conviction.

personality, fanatic (ICD: 301.0) A personality pattern dominated by overvalued ideas that are held tenaciously and may be extensively elaborated without qualifying for delusional status. Individuals may pursue their ideas combatively in defiance of social norms or adopt more private, often eccentric ways of life.

personality, hyperthymic (ICD: 301.1) A variant of **personality** characterized by cheerfulness and a high level of activity without the morbid overtones of hypomania. Hyperthymia and **dysthymia** constitute the cyclothymic personality type which is associated with **manic-depressive disease**.
See also: affective personality disorder.

personality, immature (ICD: 301.8) A **personality disorder** characterized by conduct and emotional responses that suggest a failure or lag in psychobiological development. A constitutional basis for this anomaly has been suggested by an electroencephalographic abnormality in the form of slow, paroxysmal theta or delta wave activity, mostly in the temporo-occipital areas of the brain, which is commonly associated with behavioural disorders of children and criminals. The validity of this correlation is not universally accepted.

personality, multiple (ICD: 300.1) A rare condition in which an individual exhibits two or more relatively separate, alternating **personalities. Dissociation, suggestibility,** and role-playing are all regarded as psychopathologically significant factors in the genesis of the disorder. It is usually viewed as **hysterical** but has been reported in **organic** states, especially epilepsy.

personality, passive-aggressive (ICD: 301.8) (deprecated) A **personality disorder** characterized by a pattern of aggressive feelings expressed covertly by various forms of passivity, e.g., stubbornness, sullenness, or procrastinating or inefficient behaviour.

personality, psychasthenic (ICD: 301.6) A form of **personality disorder** characterized by an asthenic physique, a low level of energy, a proneness to fatigue, lassitude, lack of conative drive, and sometimes an oversensitivity associated with obsessional traits.
Comment: The term derives from the concept of neurasthenia, introduced by Beard in 1869.
See also: dependent personality.

personality disorders (ICD: 301) Deeply ingrained maladaptive patterns of behaviour generally recognizable by the time of adolescence or earlier, and continuing throughout most of adult life, although often becoming less obvious in middle or old age. The personality is abnormal either in the balance of its components, their quality and expression or in its total aspect. Because of this deviation or **psychopathy** the patient or others suffer and there is an adverse effect on the individual or on society. It includes what is sometimes called **psychopathic personality**, but if this is determined primarily by malfunctioning of the brain, it should be classified as one of the

nonpsychotic organic brain syndromes. When the patient exhibits an anomaly of personality directly related to the neurosis or **psychosis**, e.g., **schizoid** personality and **schizophrenia** or **anankastic personality** and **obsessive-compulsive neurosis**, the relevant neurosis or psychosis which is in evidence should also be diagnosed [MDG].
Synonyms: psychopathic personality; psychopathy.

personality disorder, affective (ICD: 301.1) A condition characterized by lifelong predominance of a pronounced **mood** which may be persistently depressive, persistently elated, or alternately one then the other. During periods of **elation** there is unshakeable optimism and an enhanced zest for life and activity, whereas periods of **depression** are marked by worry, pessimism, low output of energy and a sense of futility [MDG]. Such individuals are prone to **manic-depressive psychosis** but it does not occur inevitably.
Synonyms: cycloid personality; cyclothymic personality; depressive personality; dysthymic personality; hyperthymic personality.

personality disorder, anankastic (ICD: 301.4) A lifelong pattern of personality organization characterized by feelings of personal insecurity, doubt and incompleteness leading to excessive conscientiousness, stubbornness and caution. There may be insistent and unwelcome thoughts or impulses which do not attain the severity of an **obsessive-compulsive disorder**. There is perfectionism and meticulous accuracy and a need to check repeatedly in an attempt to ensure this. Rigidity and excessive doubt may be conspicuous [MDG].
Synonyms: compulsive personality, obsessional personality.

personality disorder, asthenic (ICD: 301.6) Personality disorder characterized by passivity and a weak or inadequate response to the demands of daily life. Lack of vigour may show itself in the intellectual or emotional spheres; there is little capacity for enjoyment [MDG].
Synonyms: inadequate personality; passive personality.

personality disorder, explosive (ICD: 301.3) Personality disorder characterized by instability of mood with liability to intemperate outbursts of anger, hate, violence or affection. Aggression may be expressed in words or in physical violence. The outbursts cannot readily be controlled by the affected person, who is not otherwise prone to antisocial behaviour.
Synonyms: aggressive personality; emotional instability (excessive).

personality disorder, hysterical (ICD: 301.5) A personality pattern characterized by shallow, labile affectivity, dependence on others, craving for appreciation and attention, suggestibility and theatricality. There is often sexual immaturity, e.g., frigidity, and over-responsiveness to stimuli. Under **stress** hysterical symptoms (neurosis) may develop [MDG].
Synonyms: histrionic personality; psychoinfantile personality.

personality disorder, schizoid (ICD: 301.2) Personality disorder in which there is withdrawal from affection, and social and other contacts, with **autistic** preference for fantasy and introspective reserve. Behaviour may be slightly eccentric or indicate avoidance of competitive situations. Apparent coolness and detachment may mask an incapacity to express feeling [MDG].

personality disorder with predominantly sociopathic or asocial manifestations (ICD: 301.7) Personality disorder characterized by disregard for social obligations, lack of feeling for others, and impetuous or callous unconcern. There is a gross disparity between behaviour and the prevailing social norms. Behaviour is not readily modifiable by experience, including punishment. People with this personality are often affectively cold and may be abnormally aggressive or irresponsible. Their tolerance to frustration is low; they blame others or offer plausible rationalizations for the behaviour which brings them into conflict with society [MDG].
Synonyms: amoral personality; antisocial personality disorder; asocial personality; moral insanity (deprecated); sociopathic personality.

phobic state (ICD: 300.2) Neurotic disorder with abnormally intense dread of certain objects or specific situations which would not normally have that effect. If the **anxiety** tends to spread from a specified situation or object to a wider range of circumstances, it becomes akin to or identical with an anxiety state, and should be classified as such [MDG].
See also: anxiety states.
Synonyms: phobic neurosis; phobic disorder.

physiological malfunctions arising from mental factors (ICD: 306) A variety of physical symptoms or types of physiological malfunction of mental origin, not involving tissue damage and usually mediated through the autonomic nervous system [MDG].
Synonyms: psychophysiological disorders; psychosomatic disorders.

pica of nonorganic origin (ICD: 307.5) Craving for, and eating of nonnutritive substances, such as dirt, paint, clay, plaster, or ice. This behaviour may be related to mineral deficiency (e.g., iron deficiency) but it can also occur, as a transient disorder, in children and adolescents without any associated pathology. Pica should be distinguished from the bulimic omnivorousness occurring sometimes in **infantile autism**, **schizophrenia**, and organic cerebral disorders such as **dementia**.

Pick's disease (ICD: 290.1; 331.1) A form of **presenile dementia** characterized by early, slowly progressive changes of character and social deterioration leading to impairment of intellect, memory and language functions with apathy, euphoria and, occasionally, extrapyramidal phenomena. Women are affected more than men and there may be a hereditary pattern of transmission, probably determined by an incompletely penetrant autosomal gene. The

brain suffers a generalized atrophy with circumscribed shrinkage of the frontal and temporal lobes but without the occurrence of senile plaques and neurofibrillary tangles.
Comment: The condition was first described by Pick (1851-1924).
Synonym: morbus Pick.

postconcussional syndrome (ICD: 310.2) States occurring after generalized contusion of the brain, in which the symptom picture may resemble that of the **frontal lobe syndrome** or that of any of the **neurotic disorders**, but in which in addition, headache, giddiness, fatigue, insomnia and a subjective feeling of impaired intellectual ability are usually prominent. **Mood** may fluctuate, and quite ordinary **stress** may produce exaggerated fear and apprehension. There may be marked intolerance of mental and physical exertion, undue sensitivity to noise, and **hypochondriacal** preoccupation. The symptoms are more common in people who have previously suffered from **neurotic** or **personality disorders**, or when there is a possibility of compensation. This syndrome is particularly associated with the closed type of head injury when signs of localized brain damage are slight or absent, but it may also occur in other conditions [MDG].
Synonyms: post-traumatic brain syndrome, nonpsychotic; status post commotio cerebri.

post-traumatic organic psychosis (ICD: 293.0) Most usually an acute or subacute confusional state following cerebral injury. **Epileptic psychosis** and episodes of **delirium** may be related to brain damage. **Schizophrenic, paranoid, affective** (principally hypomanic), and hysterical psychoses do occur following head injury but are rare, and occur in predisposed individuals.
Synonym: psychosis following head injury.

premenstrual tension syndrome (ICD: 625.4) A group of physical and psychological symptoms which in varying combinations characteristically recur in women in the second, luteal phase of the menstrual cycle and subside during the first 11-12 days of the cycle. The commonest symptoms include tension, **irritability, depression**, painful breasts, fluid retention and backache. The relationship of mental ill-health and hormonal disturbance to this syndrome remains unclear.
See also: psychogenic dysmenorrhoea.

pseudoschizophrenia (ICD: 295.5) (deprecated) A group of disorders resembling **schizophrenia** in some of their clinical features but belonging to different diagnostic categories. According to Rümke the 'pseudoschizophrenias' include **manic-depressive illnesses, organic** states, severe **hysterical** reactions, **obsessive-compulsive** conditions, and **schizoid** and **paranoid personality disorders**.
See also: latent schizophrenia.

psychalgia (ICD: 307.8) Cases in which there are pains of mental origin, e.g., headache or backache, when a more precise medical or psychiatric diagnosis cannot be made.
See also: tension headache.

psychasthenia (ICD: 300.8) Neurotic disorder characterized by a 'lowering of mental function', doubts, impulsions, and **phobias**, and a consequent difficulty in arriving at conclusions, decisions, beliefs, or action. Psych-asthenic states are broadly, though not completely, distinguished from **hysterical** conditions and have been attributed to an ill-defined 'lack of psychic energy'.
Comment: The term was first employed by Janet (1859-1947).
See also: psychasthenic personality disorder.
Synonym: psychasthenic neurosis.

psychic factors associated with physical conditions (ICD: 316) Mental disturbances or psychic factors of any type, thought to have played a major part in the etiology of physical conditions, usually involving tissue damage, classified outside Chapter V of ICD-9. The mental disturbance is usually mild and nonspecific and psychic factors (worry, fear, conflict, etc.) may be present without any overt psychiatric disorder. In rare instances an overt psychiatric disorder may have caused a physical condition [MDG].

psychogenic cyclical vomiting (ICD: 306.4) Sudden attacks of vomiting in children, which, in the absence of gastrointestinal disease, last for several days and cease abruptly, with a tendency to recur after intervals of several weeks or longer. Emotional difficulties are thought to underlie the disturbance.

psychogenic dysmenorrhoea (ICD: 306.5) Abdominal pain or cramps occurring during menstruation (and not as part of the premenstrual tension syndrome), for which underlying psychological causes have been postulated without being convincingly demonstrated.
See also: premenstrual tension syndrome.

psychogenic hiccough, psychogenic cough (ICD: 306.1) Hiccough (singultus), the involuntary spasm of the inspiratory muscles followed by an abrupt closure of the glottis, can be a normal transient occurrence after eating or drinking or, when persisting or recurring frequently, a symptom of a somatic disease. **Psychogenic** causation has been surmised, but not proved, in cases where no physical cause is found. In contrast, a dry, unproductive cough in the absence of respiratory or central nervous system disease, is more readily accepted to be a neurotic symptom or an isolated psychogenic **tic**.

psychogenic pruritus (ICD: 306.3) Severe, continual, or recurrent, itching in the absence of pre-existing skin lesions. The patient seeks relief in deep, persistent scratching which may result in factitious lesions but, typically, no pain is reported. Suppressed emotional tension has been invoked as the underlying mechanism, but before such etiology is assumed, other possibilities, especially certain slowly progressing disorders like primary biliary cirrhosis, should be ruled out.

psychogenic torticollis (ICD: 306.0) Dyskinetic movements of neck muscles resulting in abnormal and often painful postures of the head. The pathophysiology of the disorder is poorly understood. **Psychogenic** etiology has been suspected for the isolated occurrence of the symptom, without associated vertebral or ocular signs, and in the absence of neurological disease, such as dystonia musculorum deformans.

psychoneurosis (ICD: 300.9) (deprecated) A term used by Freud in the early formulations of psychoanalytical theory to denote **neurotic disorders (conversion hysteria, obsessive-compulsive neurosis)** thought to arise as manifestations or representations of early traumatic experiences, in contrast to 'actual' neuroses **(neurasthenia, anxiety neurosis)** where the symptoms were regarded as direct products of thwarted libido. The distinction subsequently lost its importance in psychoanalytical thinking, and the term became a mere synonym of 'neurosis'.
See also: neurotic disorders.

psychopathy, psychopathic personality (ICD: 301.9) Terms, introduced by·Koch in 1891, which have become widely used with reference to a poorly defined group of abnormal **personalities** who either suffer personally because of their abnormality or make the community suffer because of it. While the German school of psychiatrists has tended to emphasize the biological aspects of psychopathy as not so much an illness as a statistical deviation from a hypothetical norm, Anglo-Saxon workers have stressed its social implications, especially the antisocial conduct which is often a prominent feature. There is also increasing evidence of lesional etiology.
See also: personality disorders.

psychosis (ICD: 290-299) An inexact term introduced by von Feuchtersleben in 1846, and subsequently applied to a heterogeneous group of conditions that have in common a severe impairment of mental functioning (excluding **mental retardation**) associated with disordered psychological contact with reality and, usually, aberrant social behaviour. Disorders of **consciousness**, memory, **mood**, perception, thinking or **psychomotor** behaviour are prominent clinical phenomena depending on the nature of the psychosis, and **insight** is often grossly deficient. The adjectival form, 'psychotic', is often used in a purely descriptive sense to indicate the presence of certain symptoms like delusions, hallucinations, and thought disorder. From an etiological point of view the psychoses are generally subdivided into those with manifest physical disease affecting cerebral functions (the **organic** psychoses) and those with undetermined structural or metabolic pathology (the functional or '**endogenous**' psychoses).

psychosocial dwarfism (ICD: 316, 259.4) Stunted growth and failure to thrive in childhood which are reversible and have been attributed to the psychological effects of distortions of the parent—child relationship. The evidence for a primary psychological causation is now disputed, and inadequate food intake, usually masked by psychosocial problems in the family, is thought to be the principal factor.
Synonym: deprivation dwarfism.

psychosomatic disorders (ICD: 306, 316) An ill-defined term with holistic overtones and dualistic assumptions which has been applied principally to conditions in which emotional disturbances play a significant part in the causation, aggravation or maintenance of the morbid physical process characterizing the disease. The 'psychosomatic' concept is overextensive and should be used more specifically if it is to be retained.
See also: physiological malfunction arising from mental factors.

psychosis, reactive (ICD: 298) A term employed to designate a group of **psychoses** causally related to a preceding external event, e.g., personal loss, bereavement, insult, natural disaster. The psychoses are mostly of brief duration, often but not always remitting with the recession of the provoking factor. Their form and content tend to reflect the nature of the precipitant and to fall into three broad clinical categories: disorders of consciousness (**confusional**), disorders of affect (**depression**), and delusional disorders (**paranoid**). This classification of the reactive psychoses, originally delineated by Wimmer (1916) as **psychogenic** psychoses, is widely but not universally accepted. In ICD-9, the term refers to a small group of psychotic conditions that are largely or entirely attributable to a recent life experience [MDG]. The term should not be used for the wider range of psychoses in which environmental factors play some (but not the major) part in etiology.
Synonym: psychogenic psychosis.

psychosis, reactive, depressive type (ICD: 298.0) A depressive **psychosis** which can be similar in its symptoms to **manic-depressive psychosis**, depressed type, but is apparently provoked by a saddening **stress** such as bereavement, or a severe disappointment or frustration. Compared with manic-depressive psychosis, depressed type, there may be less clinical variation of symptoms and the **delusions** are more often understandable in the context of the life experiences. There is usually a serious disturbance of behaviour, e.g., major suicidal attempt [MDG].
Synonyms: reactive depressive psychosis; psychogenic depressive psychosis.

psychosis, reactive, excitative type (ICD: 291.1) An affective psychosis similar to **manic-depressive psychosis**, manic type, but apparently provoked by emotional **stress** [MDG].

reading retardation, specific (ICD: 315.0) Disorders in which the main feature is a serious impairment in the development of reading or spelling **skills** which is not explicable in terms of general **mental retardation** or of inadequate schooling. Speech or language difficulties, impaired right-left differentiation, perceptuomotor problems, and coding difficulties are frequently associated. Similar problems are often present in other members of the family. Adverse psychosocial factors may be present [MDG].
Synonyms: developmental dyslexia; specific spelling difficulty; legasthenia; developmental reading disorder (DSM-III).

relationship problems (ICD: 313.3) Emotional disorders characteristic of childhood in which the main symptoms involve relationship problems, e.g., sibling jealousy.

sadism (ICD: 302.8) After Marquis de Sade (1740-1814), the experience of sexual excitement and gratification from inflicting pain or humiliation on another person.

schizophrenia, atypical (ICD: 295.8) A group of conditions, with a variable schizophrenic symptomatology, an episodic course with remissions, and a heavy genetic loading. According to Leonhard, atypical or 'nonsystematic' schizophrenia can be subdivided into three varieties: affect-laden paraphrenia, schizophasia, and periodic catatonia. The nosological status of these illnesses remains undecided.
Comment: The concept was introduced by Kleist (1879-1960).

schizophrenia, childhood type (ICD: 299.9) A schizophrenic **psychosis** with an onset in preadolescence or childhood (but very rarely before the age of 7), more common in boys, which usually exhibits all the major features of the disorder seen in adults. For a long time the term 'childhood schizophrenia' has been used as a collective term for all psychotic disorders in childhood; clearly, this extended usage of the term should be abandoned.
Synonyms: schizophrenia with onset in childhood (preferred); childhood schizophrenia (deprecated); dementia praecocissima (deprecated); schizophrenic syndrome of childhood.

schizophrenia, coenesthopathic (ICD: 295.8) (deprecated) A chronic state of general physical ill-being characterized by abnormal sensations in various parts of the body and not attributable to any identifiable morbid process. When coenestopathia constitutes a feature of the schizophrenias, delusional interpretation is prominent. The term was introduced in 1907 by Dupré (1862-1921). As a diagnostic entity coenestopathic schizophrenia is no longer generally accepted and the continued use of the term is not recommended.

schizophrenia, latent (ICD: 295.5) (deprecated) A term introduced by Bleuler (1911) to designate a cluster of abnormal personality traits which he attributed to an underlying schizophrenic process though positive evidence of schizophrenia was lacking. Closely related concepts are 'borderline' schizophrenia and the 'schizotypal' personality disorder. In ICD-9, the term is not recommended for general use but a description is provided for those who believe it to be useful: 'a condition of eccentric or inconsequent behaviour and anomalies of affect which give the impression of schizophrenia though no definite and characteristic schizophrenic anomalies, present or past, have been manifest' [MDG].
Synonyms: borderline schizophrenia; pseudoneurotic schizophrenia; pseudo-psychopathic schizophrenia; schizotypal personality disorder; schizophrenia larvata.

schizophrenia, paraphrenic (ICD: 295.3) A term applied occasionally to **paranoid** schizophrenic illnesses of relatively late onset in which the clinical picture is dominated by **systematized** expansive or fantastic **delusions.** In Leonhard's schema **paraphrenia** is the preferred term for all paranoid forms of schizophrenic psychosis within the 'systematic' group of the disorder.

schizophrenia, prepsychotic (ICD: 295.5) A phase that precedes the onset of a schizophrenic illness and in which the patient deviates from the premorbid state without exhibiting the characteristic symptoms of the illness.
Synonym: prodromal schizophrenia.

schizophrenia, residual (ICD: 295.6) A chronic form of schizophrenia in which the symptoms that persist from the acute phase have mostly lost their sharpness. Emotional response is blunted and thought disorder, even when gross, does not prevent the accomplishment of routine work [MDG].
Synonyms: chronic undifferentiated schizophrenia; Restzustand (schizophrenic); schizophrenic residual state; schizophrenic defect state.

schizophrenic episode, acute (ICD: 295.4) Schizophrenic disorders, in which there is a **dream-like** state with slight **clouding of consciousness** and **perplexity**. External things, people and events may become charged with personal significance for the patient. There may be ideas of reference and emotional turmoil. In many such cases **remission** occurs within a few weeks or months, even without treatment [MDG].
See also: bouffée délirante and oneirophrenia.
Synonym: acute schizophreniform psychosis.

schizophrenic psychoses (ICD: 295) A group of psychoses in which there is a fundamental disturbance of **personality**, a characteristic distortion of

thinking, often a sense of being controlled by alien forces, **delusions** which may be bizarre, disturbed perception, abnormal affect out of keeping with the real situation, and **autism**. Nevertheless, clear **consciousness** and intellectual capacity are usually maintained. The disturbance of personality involves its most basic functions which give normal people their feelings of individuality, uniqueness and self-direction. The most intimate thoughts, feelings and acts are often felt to be known to or shared by others and explanatory delusions may develop, to the effect that natural or supernatural forces are at work to influence the schizophrenic person's thoughts and actions in ways that are often bizarre. The patient may see him or herself as the pivot of all that happens. **Hallucinations**, especially of hearing, are common and may comment on, or address, the patient. Perception is frequently disturbed in other ways; there may be **perplexity**, irrelevant features may become all-important and, accompanied by passivity feelings, may lead the patient to believe that everyday objects and situations possess a special, usually sinister, meaning intended for him or her. In the characteristic schizophrenic disturbance of thinking, peripheral and irrelevant features of a total concept, which are inhibited in normal directed mental activity, are brought to the forefront and utilized in place of the elements relevant and appropriate to the situation. Thus thinking becomes vague, elliptical and obscure, and its expression in speech sometimes incomprehensible. Breaks and interpolations in the flow of consecutive thought are frequent, and the patient may be convinced that his or her thoughts are being withdrawn by some outside agency. Mood may be shallow, capricious or incongruous. Ambivalence and disturbance of volition may appear as inertia, **negativism** or **stupor**. **Catatonia** may be present. The diagnosis 'schizophrenia' should not be made unless there is, or has been evident during the same illness, characteristic disturbance of thought, perception, mood, conduct, or personality – preferably in at least two of these areas. The diagnosis should not be restricted to conditions running a protracted, deteriorating, or chronic course [MDG].
Synonyms: schizophrenia; schizophrenic disorders.

schizophrenic psychosis, catatonic type (ICD: 295.2) Includes as an essential feature prominent **psychomotor disturbances** often alternating between extremes such as hyperkinesis and **stupor**, or **automatic obedience** and **negativism**. Constrained attitudes may be maintained for long periods: if the patient's limbs are put in some unnatural position they may be held there for some time after the external force has been removed. Severe excitement may be a striking feature of the condition. Depressive or hypomanic concomitants may be present [MDG].
Synonym: catatonic schizophrenia.

schizophrenic psychosis, hebephrenic type (ICD: 295.1) A form of **schizophrenia** in which affective changes are prominent. **Delusions** and

hallucinations fleeting and fragmentary, behaviour irresponsible and un-predictable and **mannerisms** are common. The **mood** is shallow and in-appropriate, accompanied by giggling or self-satisfied, self-absorbed smiling, or by a lofty manner, grimaces, mannerisms, pranks, hypochondriacal complaints and reiterated phrases. Thought is disorganized. There is a tendency to remain solitary, and behaviour seems empty of purpose and feeling. This form of schizophrenia usually starts between the ages of 15 and 25 years [MDG].
Synonyms: hebephrenic schizophrenia; hebephrenia.

schizophrenic psychosis, paranoid type (ICD: 295.3) The form of schizophrenia in which relatively stable **delusions**, which may be accompanied by **hallucinations**, dominate the clinical picture. The delusions are frequently of persecution but may take other forms (for example of jealousy, exalted birth, Messianic mission or bodily change). Hallucinations and erratic behaviour may occur; in some cases conduct is seriously disturbed from the outset, thought disorder may be gross, and **affective flattening** with frag-mentary delusions and hallucinations may develop [MDG].
Synonym: paranoid schizophrenia.

schizophrenic psychosis, schizoaffective type (ICD: 295.7) A psy-**chosis** in which pronounced **manic** or **depressive** features are intermingled with **schizophrenic** features and which tends towards remission without permanent **defect**, but which is prone to recur. The diagnosis should be made only when both the affective and schizophrenic symptoms are pronounced [MDG].
Synonyms: cyclic schizophrenia; periodic schizophrenia; mixed schizo-
           phrenic and affective psychosis; schizoaffective psychosis;
           schizophreniform psychosis, affective type.

schizophrenic psychosis, simple type (ICD: 295.0) (deprecated) A **psychosis** in which there is insidious development of oddities of conduct, inability to meet the demands of society, and decline in total performance. **Delusions** and **hallucinations** are not in evidence and the condition is less obviously psychotic than are the **hebephrenic**, **catatonic** and **paranoid** types of schizophrenia. With increasing social impoverishment vagrancy may ensue and the patient may become self-absorbed, idle and aimless [MDG].
Synonym: schizophrenia simplex.

schizophreniform psychosis (ICD: 295.4, 295.7, 295.9, 298.8) A group of disorders with some **schizophrenic** features and a relatively benign course. Characteristically the schizophrenic symptoms are accessory rather than fundamental (in the sense of Bleuler) and the clinical picture is often dominated by **delusions, hallucinations**, and disturbances of either **conscious-ness (confusional** type) or affect (**affective** type). The onset is usually acute and the duration short. The term was introduced by Langfeldt in 1939. The validity of the concept is not universally accepted. In DSM-III, schizo-phreniform psychosis is merely a schizophrenic illness of less than six months' but more than two weeks' duration.

sensitive delusion of reference (ICD: 297.8) A particular form of nonschizophrenic **paranoid psychosis** with morbid ideas of self-reference, arising on the basis of an introverted 'sensitive' character structure with a poorly developed capacity for discharging affect and tension. The psychosis usually follows a significant experience involving humiliation and wounded self-esteem. The personality is characteristically well-preserved and the prognosis is favourable.
Comment: The concept was introduced by Kretschmer (1888-1964) as 'sensitiver Beziehungswahn'.

sexual deviations and disorders (ICD: 302) Abnormal sexual incli-nations or behaviour which are part of a referral problem. The limits and features of normal sexual inclination and behaviour have not been stated absolutely in different societies and cultures but are broadly such as serve approved social and biological purposes. The sexual activity of affected people is directed primarily towards sexual acts not normally associated with coitus, or towards coitus performed under abnormal circumstances. If the anomalous behaviour becomes manifest only during psychosis or other mental illness the condition should be seen as secondary to it. It is common for more than one anomaly to occur together in the same individual. It is preferable not to include in this category individuals who perform deviant sexual acts when normal sexual outlets are not available to them [MDG].

simple disturbance of activity and attention in childhood (ICD: 314.0) Cases in which short attention span, distractibility, and overactivity are the main manifestations of a **hyperkinetic syndrome** without significant dis-turbance of conduct or delay in acquiring specific **skills** [MDG].
Synonym: overactivity.

sleep disorders, specific (ICD: 307.4) In ICD-9, a category including nonorganic sleep disorders like hypersomnia, **insomnia**, inversion of sleep rhythm, nightmares, night terrors, and **sleep-walking**, for which a more precise medical or psychiatric diagnosis cannot be made [MDG].

sleep-walking (ICD: 307.4) A state of automatism occurring in the course of normal sleep, most commonly in childhood, and sometimes related to emotional disturbance. Episodes of sleep-walking are characterized by repetitive and purposeless movements with a low level of awareness and critical skill which can lead to self-injury; there is complete **amnesia** for the

events subsequently. The incidents occur during sleep stages 3 and 4 but not during rapid-eye-movement (REM) sleep.
Synonym: somnambulism.

stammering and stuttering (ICD: 307.0) Disorders in the rhythm of speech, in which the individual knows precisely what he or she wishes to say, but at the time is unable to say it because of an involuntary, repetitive prolongation or cessation of a sound [MDG].
Synonyms: logoneurosis (deprecated); logospasm.

stereotyped repetitive movements (ICD: 307.3) Disorders in which voluntary repetitive stereotyped movements, which are not due to any psychiatric or neurological condition, constitute the main feature. Includes head-banging, **spasmus nutans**, rocking, twirling, finger-flicking **mannerisms**, and eye poking. Such movements are particularly common in cases of **mental retardation** with sensory impairment or with environmental monotony [MDG].

symptomatic psychosis (ICD: 293) A physically induced, usually short-lived psychotic state accompanying infections, systemic, visceral and endocrine disease, and pregnancy and the puerperium. The clinical features are most often those of **clouded consciousness**, a dysmnesic state, **depression**, or **psychomotor excitement**, but syndromes resembling closely the 'functional' psychoses have also been described. Causal factors can include metabolic and toxic disturbances and a constitutional predisposition. In ICD-9, an additional code is used to identify the associated physical or neurological condition.
Synonym: transient organic psychotic conditions.

teeth grinding (ICD: 306.8) Habitual clenching or grinding of the teeth, unrelated to mastication, and occurring in either sleep or the waking state. The subject usually lacks full awareness of the symptom. The causes can be multiple but release of emotional tension through muscular contractions is commonly implicated.
Synonym: bruxism.

tension headache (ICD: 300.5, 307.8) A sensation of tightness, pressure, or dull pain which may be generalized or, more typically, have a 'band-like' quality. As a transient disturbance, it is commonly associated with the **stresses** of everyday life but, when persistent, may be a presenting feature of an **anxiety state** or a **depressive** illness.

tics (ICD: 307.2) Disorders of no known organic origin in which the outstanding feature consists of quick, involuntary, apparently purposeless, and frequently repeated movements which are not due to any neurological condition. Any part of the body may be involved but the face is most

frequently affected. Only one form of tic may be present, or there may be a combination of tics which are carried out simultaneously, alternatively or consecutively [MDG].
See also: Gilles de la Tourette syndrome.

tobacco abuse (ICD: 305.1) Cases in which tobacco is used to the detriment of a person's health or social functioning or in which there is tobacco dependence [MDG].
Synonym: tobacco dependence.

Wernicke encephalopathy (ICD: 291.1) An acute or subacute syndrome presenting characteristically with **confusion**, ophthalmoplegia, and ataxia. These phenomena may occur together or in various combinations and with prodromal anorexia, nausea and vomiting, peripheral neuropathy, malnutrition, lethargy, hypotension, memory disorders, **delirium** and emotional disturbances. The neuropathology is of bilateral symmetrical necrosis of nerve cells, gliosis, demyelination, endothelial proliferation, and petechial haemorrhages affecting chiefly the regions of the third and fourth ventricles and aqueduct, involving especially the mamillary bodies, terminal fornices, and hypothalamus. The syndrome results from a deficiency of thiamine and is associated with several clinical conditions, especially chronic **alcohol dependence** but also gastric ulcer and carcinoma, pernicious anaemia, dietary insufficiences, persistent vomiting, and pregnancy. It is closely related to beriberi and to **Korsakov's syndrome**. The response to early thiamine administration is good, but severe cases tend to exhibit residual defects even after treatment. The condition was first described by Wernicke (1848-1905) in 1881.
See also: Korsakov's psychosis.
Synonyms: Wernicke's disease; polioencephalitis haemorrhagica superior; Gayet-Wernicke syndrome; breast milk intoxication (deprecated); encephalopathia alcoholica; cerebral beriberi.

writer's cramp (ICD: 300.8) A painful spasm of the muscles of the hand and the fingers used in writing, which appears at the start or shortly after the beginning of the writing act, and tends to recur.
See also: occupational neurosis.
Synonyms: graphospasm; scrivener's palsy (deprecated).

Part II

Names for symptoms and signs

Names of symptoms or signs of disorders and other psychopathological terms used in the description or definition of various diseases, syndromes and conditions

aerophagy (ICD: 306.4) Habitual swallowing of air, with resulting abdominal distension and eructations, often accompanied by **hyperventilation**. It can occur in the context of **hysteria** and **anxiety** states, but also as a monosymptomatic manifestation.

affect, abnormal (ICD: 295) A general term describing morbid, or unusual mood-states, of which the most common are **depression, anxiety, elation, irritability**, and **affective lability**.
See also: affective flattening; affective psychosis; anxiety; depression; mood, disturbance of; elation; emotion; mood; schizophrenic psychoses.

affect, lability of (ICD: 290-294) The uncontrolled, unstable, fluctuating expression of emotions, encountered most frequently in organic brain syndromes, early **schizophrenia** and some forms of **neurotic** and **personality disorders**.
See also: mood, fluctuation of.

affect, shallowness of (ICD: 295) A state of morbid insufficiency of emotional response, presenting as an indifference to external events and situations, occurring characteristically in **schizophrenia** of the **hebephrenic** type but also in **organic** cerebral disorders, **mental retardation**, and **personality disorders**.

affective flattening (ICD: 295.3) Observable disturbance of affective response and variety, expressed as emotional blunting and indifference, especially as a symptom occurring in **schizophrenic psychoses**, organic **dementia**, or **psychopathic personality**.
Synonyms: emotional blunting; affective dullness.

aggressiveness, aggression (ICD: 301.3, 301.7, 309.3, 310.0) As a biological feature of infrahuman organisms, aggressiveness is a component of animal behaviour which is released in particular conditions, for the satisfaction of vital needs, and for the elimination of environmental threat, but not for destructive purposes unless these are related to predatory activity. In humans the concept is widened to incorporate harmful behaviour, normal or morbid, directed against others or the self, and motivated by hostility, anger or competitiveness.

agitation (ICD: 296.1) Marked restlessness and excessive motor activity, accompanied by **anxiety**.

agitation, catatonic (ICD: 295.2) A state in which the psychomotor features of anxiety are associated with catatonic syndromes.

ambitendence (ICD: 295.2) A **psychomotor disturbance** characterized by an **ambivalence** towards a voluntary action, leading to contradictory behaviour. The phenomenon is most frequently exhibited in the **catatonic** syndrome in **schizophrenia**.

ambivalence (ICD: 295) The coexistence of contradictory emotions, ideas or wishes concerning the same person, object or situation. According to Bleuler, who introduced the term in 1910, transient ambivalence is part of normal mental life; in its severe or persistent form it is a primary symptom of **schizophrenia**, where it may be affective, ideational, or volitional. It is also a feature of **obsessive-compulsive disorder** and is sometimes seen in **manic-depressive psychoses**, especially in retarded depression.

amnesia, selective (ICD: 300.1) A form of **psychogenic** memory loss restricted to associations of the psychological precipitant of the reaction which is usually classified as **hysterical**.

anhedonia (ICD: 300.5, 301.6) An absence of the capacity to experience pleasure, associated most frequently with some **schizophrenic** and **depressive** states.
Comment: The concept was introduced by Ribot (1839-1916).

anxiety (ICD: 292.1, 296, 300, 308.0, 309.2, 313.0) In its morbid connotation a subjectively unpleasant emotional state of fear or apprehension directed towards the future, either in the absence of any recognizable threat or danger, or when such factors are clearly out of keeping with the reaction. Subjective bodily discomfort and manifest voluntary and autonomic bodily dysfunction may accompany the anxiety. Anxiety may be situational or specific, i.e., tied to some particular situation or object, or 'free-floating', when no such link to an external triggering factor is apparent. Trait anxiety may be distinguished from state anxiety, the former referring to an enduring aspect of personality structure and the latter to a temporary disorder.
Comment: The translation of the English term 'anxiety' into other languages may present particular difficulties because of subtle differences in connotation exhibited by words that refer to the same basic concept.

astasia-abasia (ICD: 300.1) Incoordination in the erect position, and a resulting inability to stand or walk, with intact capacity for leg movements while sitting or lying down. In the absence of an **organic** lesion to the central nervous system, astasia-abasia is usually a manifestation of **hysteria**. Astasia, however, can also be a sign of organic cerebral pathology, especially involving the frontal lobes or corpus callosum.

autism (ICD: 295) A term introduced by Bleuler to designate a form of thinking characterized by a turning away from reality, uncommunicativeness, and an excessive indulgence in fantasy. Pervasive autism, according to Bleuler, is a fundamental symptom of **schizophrenia**. The term is also employed to label a specific form of childhood psychosis.
See also: autism, infantile.

automatic obedience (ICD: 295.2) The phenomenon of undue compliance with instructions, a feature of 'command automatism' associated with **catatonic** syndromes and the hypnotic state.

catalepsy (ICD: 295.2) A morbid state, of sudden onset and lasting for brief or long periods, in which voluntary movement and sensibility are suspended. Limbs and body may exhibit a waxy rigidity (**flexibilitas cerea**) and maintain externally imposed postures. Respiration and pulse are slowed, and body temperature falls. A distinction is sometimes made between flexible and rigid catalepsy. In the former the posture is assumed at the slightest external prompting; in the latter, the posture is resistent to external attempts at modification. The condition may be associated with organic cerebral disease (e.g., encephalitis), **catatonic schizophrenia**, **hysteria** and hypnosis.
Synonyms: waxy flexibility; flexibilitas cerea.

catatonia (ICD: 295.2) A range of qualitative psychomotor and volitional disturbances including **stereotypies, mannerisms, automatic obedience, catalepsy,** echokinesis and echopraxia, **mutism, negativism**, automatisms and impulsive acts. These phenomena may occur against a background of hyperkinesis, hypokinesis, or akinesis. Catatonia was described as a separate disease by Kahlbaum in 1874, but later subsumed by Kraepelin as one of the subtypes of dementia praecox (**schizophrenia**). Catatonic phenomena are not limited to schizophrenic psychoses and may occur in organic cerebral disease (e.g., encephalitis), other physical disease, and affective illness.

claustrophobia (ICD: 300.2) A morbid fear of confined places or spaces.
See also: agoraphobia.

compulsion (ICD: 300.3, 312.2) A powerful urge to act or behave in a way which the subject recognizes as irrational or senseless and which he or she attributes to subjective necessity rather than to external influences. When subordinate to obsession the term refers to an act or behaviour resulting from **obsessional ideas**.
See also: obsessional action.

confabulation (ICD: 291.1, 294.0) A disorder of memory in a setting of clear **consciousness,** characterized by false accounts of past events or personal experiences. The false memories are usually loosely held and have to be evoked; less commonly they are spontaneous and sustained, and occasionally tend to grandiosity. Confabulation usually occurs in **organically** based **amnestic** syndromes (e.g., Korsakov's syndrome). It can also be induced or influenced iatrogenically. It should not be confounded with the **hallucinations** of memory occurring in **schizophrenia**, or with pseudologia phantastica (Delbrück's syndrome).

confusion (ICD: 290-294) A term usually employed to designate a state of impaired **consciousness** associated with acute or chronic cerebral **organic** disease. Clinically it is characterized by **disorientation**, slowness of mental processes with scanty association of ideas, apathy, lack of initiative, fatigue, and poor attention. In mild **confusional** states, rational responses and behaviour may be provoked by examination but more severe degrees of the disorder render the subject unable to retain contact with the environment. The term is also employed loosely to describe disordered thinking in the functional psychoses: this latter usage is not recommended.
See also: confusion, reactive; consciousness, clouded.
Synonym: confusional state.

consciousness, clouded (ICD: 290-294, 295.4) A state of impaired consciousness representing mild stages of disturbance on the continuum from full awareness to coma. Disorders of awareness, orientation and perception are associated with cerebral or other physical organic disease. Although the term has been employed to cover a wider range (including the restricted perceptual field following acute emotional stress) it is best used to designate the early stages of an organically determined confusional state.
See also: confusion; consciousness.

consciousness, narrowing (restriction) of the field of (ICD: 300.1) A form of disordered consciousness in which the field is restricted to and dominated by a small group of ideas and emotions to the virtual exclusion of other content. This condition occurs in extreme fatigue and **hysteria**; it also may be associated with some forms of cerebral disorders, especially the **twilight states** of epilepsy.
See also: consciousness; consciousness, clouded; twilight state.

defect (ICD: 295.7) (deprecated) A lasting and irreversible impairment of any particular psychological function (e.g., 'cognitive defect'), of the general development of mental capacities ('mental defect'), or of the characteristic pattern of thought, feeling and behaviour constituting the individual **personality**. A defect in any one of these areas can be either innate or acquired. A characteristic defect state of the personality, ranging in its manifestations from loss of intellectual and emotional vigour, or mild eccentricities of behaviour, to autistic withdrawal or affective blunting, has been held by Kraepelin (1856-1926) and Bleuler (1857-1939) to be a hallmark of the outcome of **schizophrenic** illnesses (see also: personality change), in contradistinction from **manic-depressive** psychosis. The ubiquity of outcome into defect in the schizophrenic disorders is not supported by more recent research, nor is its irreversibility.

delinquent act (ICD: 312.2) Antisocial action by children or young people, mostly offences against property and larceny, but also including violent and sexual crimes, truancy from school, early drinking and drug abuse, and, generally, refusal to conform to social rules.
See also: delinquency.

delusion (ICD: 290-299) A false, incorrigible conviction or judgement, out of keeping with reality, and with the socially shared beliefs of the individual's background and culture. Primary delusions are essentially incomprehensible in terms of the individual's life history and personality; secondary delusions are psychologically comprehensible and arise from morbid and other states of mind, e.g., affective disorders, and suspicion. A distinction was made by Birnbaum (1908), and later elaborated by Jaspers (1913), between delusion proper and delusion-like ideas; the latter are merely mistaken judgements held with exaggerated tenacity.

delusion of bodily change A morbid belief in physical change or disease, often of a bizarre nature, and based on somatic sensations which lead to **hypochondriacal** preoccupations. The syndrome is most commonly associated with **schizophrenia** but may occur in severe **depressive** states and cerebral **organic** conditions.

delusion, explanatory (ICD: 295) A term introduced by Bleuler (Erklärungswahn) for delusional ideas that constitute quasilogical reasons for other, more generalized delusions.

delusion of grandeur A morbid belief in self-importance, greatness or superiority (e.g., **delusion of messianic mission**) often accompanied by other fantastic delusional ideas, which can be a symptom of **paranoia, schizophrenia** (often, but not invariably of the **paranoid** type), **mania**, and cerebral **organic** states, especially general paresis.
See also: grandiose ideas.

delusion of messianic mission (ICD: 295.3) Delusional conviction of being divinely chosen or destined for grandiose deeds of salvation or redemption in respect of mankind or in respect of a particular nation, religious group, etc. Messianic delusions may occur in **schizophrenia, paranoia,** and **manic-depressive psychosis** as well as in psychotic states associated with epilepsy. In some instances, especially in the absence of other overt psychotic features, they may be difficult to distinguish from the subcultural beliefs of special mission or purpose shared by members of certain fundamentalist religious sects or movements.

delusion of nihilism A form of delusion, exhibited principally in severe **depressive** states and characterized by negative ideas relating to the individual or the environment, e.g., that the outside world is nonexistent, or that the patient's bodily functions have ceased.

delusion of persecution A morbid belief in victimization by one or more individuals or groups. It occurs in **paranoid** conditions, most commonly **schizophrenia,** but also in some **depressive** and **organic** states. In certain personality disorders there is a predisposition to such delusions.

delusion of systematized kind (ICD: 297.0, 297.1) A delusional belief forming part of a coherent organization of morbid ideas. Such delusions may be primary or represent quasilogical conclusions deduced from an elaborate system of delusional premises.
Synonym: Systematized delusions.

depersonalization (ICD: 300.6) A state of disordered perception in which self-awareness becomes heightened but inanimate in the presence of a normal sensorium, and an intact capacity for emotional expression. Among a variety of complex and distressing subjective phenomena, many of them difficult to put into words, the more prominent include experience of bodily change, compulsive self-scrutiny and automatization, an absence of affective response, a disordered experience of time, and a sense of alienated identity. The subject may feel detached from his or her experiences, as though viewing himself or herself from a distance, or as if he or she were dead. **Insight** into the abnormal nature of the phenomenon is usually retained. Depersonalization may occur as an isolated phenomenon in otherwise normal people; it may accompany fatigue or an intense emotional reaction; or it may form part of the symptomatology of ruminant, **obsessional anxiety** states, **depression,** **schizophrenia**, certain personality disorders, and disorders of cerebral function. Its pathogenesis is unknown.
See also: depersonalization syndrome; derealization.

derealization (ICD: 300.6) A subjective experience of alienation similar to **depersonalization** but involving the external world rather than the subject's self-experience and personal identity. The surroundings may seem to lack colour and life and appear as artificial, or as a stage on which people are acting contrived roles.

disorientation (ICD: 290-294, 298.2) An obscuring of the temporal, topographical, or personal spheres of **consciousness,** associated with various forms of cerebral **organic** syndromes or, less commonly, with **psychogenic** disorders.

dream-like state (ICD: 295.4) A state of disordered **consciousness** in which **depersonalization** and **derealization** phenomena appear against a background

of mild **clouding of consciousness**. Dream-like states can be a step on a scale of deepening **organic** disturbances of consciousness leading to **twilight states** and **delirium**; however, they also occur in **neurotic** illness and in states of fatigue. A complex form of dream-like state with vivid, scenic visual **hallucinations** which may be accompanied by hallucinations in other sensory modalities (oneiroid (dream-like) state), may appear in epilepsy and in certain acute psychotic illnesses.
See also: oneirophrenia.

dysphoria An unpleasant mood-state characterized by disaffection, dejection, restlessness, **anxiety** and **irritability**.
See also: neurotic disorders.

dysthymia A less severe **depressive** mood-state than dysphoria associated with **neurasthenic** and **hypochondriacal** symptoms. In abnormal psychology the term is also used to refer to a cluster of **affective** and **obsessional** symptoms in individuals with a high degree of neuroticism and introversion.
See also: hyperthymic personality; neurotic disorders.

echolalia (ICD: 299.8) An automatic repetition of an interlocutor's words or phrases. It may be a feature of early normal speech development or be associated with several morbid conditions, including dysphasia, **catatonic** states, **mental retardation, autism (infantile)** and in the form of delayed echolalia.

elation (ICD: 296.0) An affective state of joyous gaiety which, when intensified and out of keeping with life circumstances, is a dominant symptom of **mania** and hypomania.
Synonym: hyperthymia.

emotion (ICD: 295, 298, 300, 308, 309, 310, 312, 313) A complex state of arousal compounded of widespread physiological changes, heightened perception and subjective experience, tending towards action.
See also: affect, abnormal; mood.

excitation, catatonic (ICD: 295.2) A state of psychomotor overactivity associated with catatonic symptoms.

fear (ICD: 291.0, 308.0, 309.2) A primitive, intense emotion in the face of threat, real or imagined, which is accompanied by physiological reactions resulting from arousal of the sympathetic nervous system and by defensive patterns of behaviour associated with avoidance, flight or concealment.

flight of ideas (ICD: 296.0) A disordered form of thinking associated commonly with manic or hypomanic mood and often experienced subjectively as pressure of thought. Characteristically, talk is rapid and incessant; speech associations are facilitated and easily diverted and distracted by chance factors, or for no obvious reasons. Increased distractibility is a prominent feature, and rhyming and punning often occur. The flow of ideas may be too insistent for expression, resulting in a form of verbal incoherence. Synonym: fuga idearum.

fugue (ICD: 300.1) A flight or wandering, of short or long duration, from familiar surroundings in a state of altered **consciousness,** usually followed by partial or complete **amnesia** for the event. Fugues are associated with **hysteria, depressive** reactions, epilepsy, and, occasionally, cerebral damage. As **psycho-genic** reactions they are often related to escape from disagreeable situations and are then likely to be more 'orderly' than the 'disorderly' epileptic and **organic** fugue states.
See also: consciousness, narrowing (restriction) of the field of.
Synonym: wandering state.

grandiose ideas (ICD: 296.0) Exaggerated notions of capacities, pos-sessions and esteem which in delusional form are associated with **mania, schizophrenia,** and cerebral **organic** psychoses, e.g., **general paresis**.
See also: delusion of grandeur.

hallucination (ICD: 290-299) A sensory perception, of any modality, occurring in the absence of the appropriate external stimulus. In addition to the sensory modality in which they occur, hallucinations may be subdivided according to their intensity, complexity, clarity of perception, and the subjective degree of their projection into the external environment. Halluci-nations may occur in normal individuals in the half-sleeping (hypnagogic) or half-waking (hypnopompic) state. As morbid phenomena they may be symptomatic of cerebral disease, functional psychoses, and the toxic effects of drugs, each with characteristic features.

hyperkinesis (ICD: 314) Excessive, unintentional motor activity of the limbs or any part of the body, appearing spontaneously or in response to stimulation. Hyperkinesis is a feature of a variety of **organic** disorders of the central nervous system but may also appear in the absence of a demonstrable localized lesion.

hyperventilation (ICD: 306.1) A condition of longer, deeper or more rapid respiratory movements eventually leading to dizziness and cramps due to acute gaseous alkalosis. It is often **psychogenic** in nature. In addition to the carpopedal spasm and tetany, the hypocapnia may be associated with subjective phenomena, notably paraesthesiae, dizziness, light-headedness, numbness, palpitations, and apprehension. Hyperventilation is a physio-logical response to hypoxia or hypocapnia but can also occur in states of **anxiety**.

ideas of reference (ICD: 295.4, 301.0) Morbid interpretations of in-different, external phenomena as carrying personal, usually noxious, signifi-cance. They tend to occur in sensitive individuals at times of **stress** and fatigue and are generally understandable in the context of the current life-situations; however, they may constitute the precursors of **delusional** beliefs.

illusion (ICD: 291.0, 293) An erroneous apperception or interpretation of an object or sensory stimulus. Illusions are experienced by most people and do not necessarily indicate mental disorder.

impulsiveness (ICD: 310.0) A temperamental factor characterized by actions which are accomplished unexpectedly and with inadequate regard for the consequences.

insight (ICD: 290-299, 300) In general psychopathology this term refers to the patient's understanding and judgement of the nature and causation of his or her own condition, and its effects on him or herself and others. Loss of insight has been widely regarded as contributing to a diagnosis of **psychosis.** In psychoanalytical terminology this form of self-knowledge is called in-tellectual insight and is distinguished from emotional insight, which refers to the capacity to feel and apprehend the significance of 'unconscious' and symbolic factors in determining emotional disturbance.

intelligence (ICD: 290, 291, 294, 310, 315, 317) The general mental ability to overcome difficulties in new situations.

irritability (ICD: 300.5) An undue state of excitability to annoyance, impatience or anger. It may appear in states of fatigue or chronic pain, or be a clinical feature of temperamental anomalies such as advancing age, cerebral trauma, epileptic states and manic-depressive disorders.

kleptomania (ICD: 312.2) An outmoded term for a morbid, often sudden and usually irresistible impulse to steal without an apparent need. The impulse tends to recur. The objects are mostly of little or no value but may carry symbolic significance. It has been described to occur more frequently in women and to be associated with depression, neurotic illness, personality disorder or mental retardation.
Synonym: shoplifting (pathological).

judgement (ICD: 290-294) A critical evaluation of the relations between objects, situations, concepts or terms; a propositional statement of these relations. In psychophysics, it is the discernment of stimuli and their intensity.

laxative habit (ICD: 305.9) Reliance on, and abuse of purgatives as a means of controlling weight, often occurring in association with 'binge eating' in bulimia.

mannerisms (ICD: 295.1) Unusual or morbid idiosyncratic psychomotor behaviour, less persistent than **stereotypies** and more in keeping with **personality** characteristics.

memory span, reduction of (ICD: 291.1) A decrease in the number of the cognitively unconnected elements or items (normally 6-10) that can be reproduced correctly after successive presentation on one single occasion. The memory span is a measure of the short-term perceptual ability.

mood (ICD: 295, 296, 301.1, 310.2) A pervasive and sustained state of feeling which in extreme or morbid degree can dominate the subject's internal and external outlook.

mood, capricious (ICD: 295) (deprecated) Changeable, inconstant or unpredictable affective reactions.

mood, disturbance of (ICD: 296) A morbid change of affect extending beyond normal variation to subsume any of several reactions, including **depression, elation, anxiety, irritability,** and anger.
See also: affect, abnormal.

mood, fluctuation of (ICD: 310.2) A morbid unstable or labile pattern of affective response without external cause.
See also: affect, lability of.

mood, inappropriate (ICD: 295.1) Morbid affective responses that are out of keeping with external stimuli.
See also: incongruity of affect; mood, incongruous; parathymia.

mood, incongruous (ICD: 295) A discrepancy between emotions and thought-content or experience. Characteristically a symptom of **schizophrenia** but also occurring in cerebral **organic** states and some forms of **personality disorder**. Not all authorities distinguish between **inappropriate mood** and incongruous mood.
See also: incongruity of affect; mood, inappropriate; parathymia.

morbid jealousy (ICD: 291.5) A complex and painful emotional state with elements of envy, anger, and desire for possession. Sexual jealousy is a well-recognized symptom of mental disorder and can occur in association with **organic** brain disease and toxic states (see mental disorders associated with alcohol), the functional psychoses (see paranoid disorders), and **neurotic** and **personality disorders**. The dominant clinical feature may be of **delusional** beliefs of infidelity or over-readiness to assume the partner's misconduct. Social mores as well as psychological mechanisms must be taken into account when assessing the possibly morbid nature of jealousy. It is often a motive for crimes of violence, particularly by men against women.

negativism (ICD: 295.2) Contrary or oppositive behaviour or attitude. Active or command negativism denotes performance of actions which are the opposite of what is requested or expected; passive negativism signifies a morbid failure to respond positively to requests or stimuli, including active muscular resistance; inner negativism (Bleuler, 1857-1939) is behaviour in which physiological urges, e.g., eating and excretion, are not obeyed. Negativism may occur in **catatonic** states, in **organic** cerebral disorder, and in some forms of **mental retardation**.

obsessional action (ICD: 312.3) Quasi-ritual performances designed to relieve anxiety (e.g., washing the hands to cope with contamination) associated with an **obsessional idea** or urge.
See also: compulsion.

obsessional ideas (ICD: 300.3, 312.3) Unwanted ideas and thoughts that intrude, insistent ruminations, or trains of thought that are perceived to be inappropriate or nonsensical and must be resisted. They are recognized as alien to the personality, but as coming from within the self [MDG].

panic attack (ICD: 300.0, 308.0) A sudden attack of intense **fear** and alarm in which the signs and symptoms of morbid **anxiety** become dominant and are often accompanied by irrational behaviour, which may be characterized by either extreme inactivity or purposeless agitated overactivity. The attack may occur in response to sudden severe environmental threats or shocks, or arise without warning or obvious precipitants in the course of anxiety neurosis.
See also: panic disorder; panic state.

paranoid (ICD: 291.5, 292.1, 294.8, 295.3, 297, 298.3, 298.4, 301.0) A descriptive term designating either morbid dominant ideas or **delusions** of self-reference concerning one or more of several themes—most commonly persecution, love, hate, envy, jealousy, honour, litigation, grandeur, and the supernatural. It may be associated with an **organic** psychosis; a toxic reaction; a **schizophrenic** condition; an independent syndrome; a reaction to emotional **stress**; or a disorder of **personality**.
Comment: It should be noted that in the French psychiatric tradition 'paranoid' does not have the above meaning; the French language equivalents are *interprétatif, délirant* or *persécutoire*.

parathymia A **schizophrenic** distortion of mood in which the affective state is inappropriate to the patient's circumstances and/or behaviour.
See also: incongruity of affect; mood, inappropriate; mood, incongruous.

passivity feelings (ICD: 295) Morbid experiences in clear **consciousness** in which thoughts, emotions, reactions or bodily activities appear to be influenced, 'made', directed or controlled by an external agency or force, human or nonhuman. Genuine passivity feelings are characteristic of

schizophrenia, but in assessing reliably their presence, account must be taken of the educational standards, cultural background, and belief system of the subject.

perplexity (ICD: 295) A state of puzzled bewilderment in which verbal responses are desultory and disjointed, reminiscent of confusion. Its clinical associations include acute **schizophrenia**, severe **anxiety, manic – depressive** illness and the **organic** psychoses with **confusion**.

personality (ICD: 290, 295, 297.2, 301, 310) The ingrained patterns of thought, feeling and behaviour characterizing an individual's unique life-style and mode of adaptation, representing the resultant of constitutional factors, development, and social experience.

personality change An alteration in basic character traits, usually for the worse, following, or as a consequence of, physical or mental disorder.

phobia (ICD: 300.2) A morbid **fear** which may be diffused or focused on one or more objects or situations, and is out of proportion to external danger or threat. It is usually accompanied by apprehension, which may lead to avoidance of such objects or situations. In some instances it is closely related to an **obsessional** condition.
See also: phobic state.

psychomotor disturbances (ICD: 308.2) Disordered expressive motor behaviour which may occur in a great variety of neurological and psychiatric conditions; examples of psychomotor disturbances are paramimia, **tics, stupor, stereotypies, catatonia,** tremor and the dyskinesias. The term 'psycho-motor epileptic seizure' was formerly used to designate epileptic seizures characterized essentially by automatic psychomotor manifestation. It has been recommended that the term 'psychomotor epileptic seizure' be discarded in favour of 'automatic epileptic seizure'.

remission (ICD: 295.7) A state of partial or complete reduction or abatement of the symptoms and signs of a disorder.

ritualistic behaviour (ICD: 299.0) Iterative, often complex, and usually symbolic actions which may serve to enhance biological signalling functions, acquire ceremonial significance for collective religious observances, and constitute a feature of play and normal development in childhood. As a morbid phenomenon, whether consisting in an exaggeration of everyday behaviour, such as compulsive dressing or washing, or assuming more bizarre forms, it is a feature of **obsessional** disorders, **schizophrenia**, and **infantile autism**.

separation anxiety (deprecated) A loosely employed term which most often designates either the normal or a morbid reaction (alarm, distress or

fear) in a young child separated from the parent(s) or parental figure(s). The causal role of such experience in the subsequent development of mental disorder is no longer accorded significance without regard to other contributory factors. Psychoanalytical theory recognizes two forms of separation anxiety: the objective and the neurotic.

social withdrawal (ICD: 295) The retreat from social and personal contact that is commonly encountered in the early stages of **schizophrenia,** when **autistic** preoccupations lead to aloof detachment and an impaired capacity to communicate with others.

spasmus nutans (ICD: 307.3) (deprecated) (1) Rhythmic anteroposterior head movements associated with compensatory balancing movements of the trunk in the same direction, with or without extension of the upper limbs, and with nystagmus. The movements are slow and occur in series of 20 to 30 in mentally retarded subjects; they are unrelated to epilepsy.

(2) The same term is sometimes used to describe an epileptic seizure occurring in children in which the head drops to the chest, owing to a loss of tone to the neck muscles, or to a tonic spasm in flexion due to contraction of the anterior neck muscles [DE].

Synonyms: salaam tic, for (1); infantile spasm, for (2).

stereotypies (ICD: 299.1) Functionally autonomous, abnormal movements which are combined into rhythmic or complex sequences of obscure purpose. In animals and humans they occur in conditions of physical constraint and of social and sensory deprivation and can be induced by drugs, e.g., amphetamine. They include repetitive locomotion, self-mutilation, head-banging, bizarre posturing of limbs and body, and manneristic behaviour. Their clinical associations include severe **mental retardation**, congenital blindness, brain damage, and the autistic syndrome in children. In adults stereotypies may be a prominent feature of **schizophrenia**, especially the **catatonic** and the **residual** forms.

stupor (ICD: 295.2) A state characterized by **mutism,** an absence or profound diminution or blocking of voluntary movement, and psychomotor unresponsiveness; **consciousness** may be disturbed, according to the nature of the causal condition. Stuporous states occur in association with **organic** cerebral disease, **schizophrenia** (especially its **catatonic** form), **depressive** illnesses, **hysterical psychosis**, and **acute reactions to stress**.

stupor, catatonic (ICD: 295.2) A state of diminished psychomotor activity associated with catatonic symptoms.

suggestibility A state of susceptibility to the uncritical acceptance of ideas, beliefs, and patterns of behaviour expressed or shown by others. Suggestibility can be heightened by environmental conditions, drugs and hypnosis, and may be prominent in people with **hysterical** personality traits. The term 'negative suggestibility' is sometimes applied to negativistic behaviour.

tolerance Pharmacological tolerance occurs when a repeated administration of a given quantity of drug produces a decreasing effect, or when increasingly larger quantities of drug are needed for the effect obtained by the original dose. Tolerance may be innate or acquired; in the latter case it can be dispositional, pharmacodynamic or behavioural.

withdrawal symptoms (ICD: 291, 292.0) The physical and mental phenomena that occur in a period of abstinence from the ingestion of a drug on which the subject is physically dependent. The nature of the symptom-complex varies with the drug concerned and may include tremor, vomiting, abdominal pain, **fear**, **delirium** and convulsions.
Synonym: abstinence symptoms.

Part III

Terms for concepts

Terms for concepts of a higher order of abstraction which are used in the delimitation of major classes or categories of disorders, or otherwise concern the general rules and principles of classification of psychiatric conditions

adaptation (ICD: 309.9) In general, the conforming of an organism to the environment. More specifically, the term is used in the 'general adaptation syndrome' (Selye) to signify the bodily changes that occur in response to **stress**. The term **'adjustment'** is often used synonymously with 'adaptation', but the English word 'adjustment' has no precise equivalent in other languages and 'adaptation' is therefore preferred.

adjustment (ICD: 309) A state of adequate **adaptation** to the environment.

atypical In medicine a term employed to designate irregularity in the phenomena or course of a disease. In those forms of mental disorder whose basic characteristics have not been established, atypicality tends to designate a residual category with unusual clinical features.

chronic/acute/subacute When applied to morbid states these terms refer principally, though imprecisely, to duration, but the term 'acute' carries overtones of severity.

cognition (ICD: 310, 317-319) A general term covering the acquisition of knowledge by means of any of various mental processes, such as conceptualization, perception, judgement or imagination. Cognition is traditionally contrasted with conation and emotion.

comprehension The capacity for understanding or grasp, as distinct from apprehension or cognition.

conduct The psychological and physical behaviour of the individual, with special reference to the standards set by the social group to which the individual belongs. Conduct or behaviour disorders in children are mostly characterized by **aggressive** and/or antisocial features.

consciousness (ICD: 290-291, 293, 295, 298.2, 300, 308) In biological, as distinct from philosophical, discourse, a complex mental state of vigilant awareness of self and environment mediated by sensory and cognitive processes.
See also: consciousness, clouded; consciousness, narrowing (restriction) of the field of.

drive A hypothetical force, closely related to instinct, originally designating an unlearned, general system of motivation with a presumptive physiological basis. Elaborate models of drive theory, including psychoanalytical hypotheses, have not been supported experimentally.

endogenous (ICD: 296.1) A term introduced into psychiatry by Möbius in 1893 for the purposes of etiological, clinical classification to designate those mental disorders caused primarily by hereditary and constitutional factors, originating within the soma or the central nervous system. The precise meanings of endogeny and exogeny are, however, too arbitrary to justify more than a provisional distinction. For example, a brain tumour although arising within the central nervous system would give rise to an 'exogenous' mental disorder, while a psychogenic psychosis would be an 'endogenous' disorder (Jaspers, 1946). The distinction, therefore, is of mainly historical significance.

learning capacity (ICD: 290-294) The individually characteristic rate of acquisition or alteration of cognitive structures through the reception and processing of information..

organic/nonorganic A dichotomy which, when applied to disease in the strict sense distinguishes between illnesses that do, or do not, relate to body organs. More generally, it covers the presence or absence of any identifiable pathophysiological process.

organic psychosyndrome A term used generally to incorporate the various patterns of psychological dysfunction that may be associated with transient or permanent cerebral disease or damage. These include **delirium, dementia, hallucinosis, personality** change and mnestic disorders. The term was employed more narrowly by Bleuler (1857-1939) as synonymous with the **amnestic** syndrome.

orientation The current appreciation of temporal, spatial and personal relations.

psychogenic (ICD: 298, 306, 307, 316) A term used widely and loosely to indicate attribution of etiology or pathogenesis to mental, psychological or emotional factors rather than to physical causes. The term was introduced into psychiatry by Sommer in 1894.
See also: reactive.

reaction (ICD: 291.4, 292.2, 293.0, 293.1, 295.9, 296.0, 296.6, 297.9, 298.3, 300.1, 300.4, 308, 309, 313.0, 313.2) An ill-defined term which, when related to mental disorder, is employed in several ways. As a noun, 'reaction' may be no more than a synonym for 'illness', 'syndrome' or 'clinical picture' or it may designate a response to an environmental change or stressful event, physical or psychosocial. There are also two compound forms of the noun: 'reaction-type', which refers to a group of organically provoked

illnesses, e.g., the exogenous reaction-type of Bonhoeffer (1868-1949), and the psychobiological reaction-types of Meyer (1866-1950); and 'reaction-formation', which in psychoanalytical theory constitutes a form of defence against unacceptable urges.
See also: reactive.

reactive (ICD: 298.0, 298.2, 298.4, 300.4) Secondary to, resulting from, or precipitated by an identifiable event. Reactivity is an ambiguous concept, often coterminous with psychogenic, applied to those neurotic and psychotic disorders that are supposedly caused or precipitated by psychosocial factors.
See also: psychogenic; reactive psychosis; reactive depression.

reality testing (deprecated) According to psychoanalytical theory, the capacity to distinguish between internal fantasy and the reality of the external world; defects in this process result in delusions and hallucinations, and constitute the major criterion of functional psychosis.

recurrent disorder A morbid process or lesion with a natural history of repeated episodes.

skills An acquired ability to carry out more or less complex psychomotor acts in various domains, including the visuospatial, symbolic, linguistic, numeral, social, learning and specific.

stress (ICD: 308) A term introduced into human physiology by Cannon in the early 1920s to denote all physical, chemical and emotional stimuli which exceed a certain critical threshold and disrupt the equilibrium of the internal milieu of the organism. In the 'general adaptation syndrome' described by Selye (1950) the term changed its meaning and became a common denominator for the nonspecific responses of the organism to such stimuli. In current usage it is used interchangeably to describe various aversive stimuli of excessive intensity; the physiological, behavioural and subjective responses to them; the context mediating the encounter between the individual and the stressful stimuli; or all of the above as a 'system'. The term is clearly overstretched and should be used sparingly.

List of technical advisors

The following individuals have contributed comments and suggestions, or otherwise assisted at various stages of the preparation of this lexicon.

Dr K. Achté (Helsinki, Finland), Dr T. A. Baasher (Khartoum, Sudan), Dr Z. Bankowski, (CIOMS, Geneva, Switzerland), Dr J. Barahona Fernandes (Lisbon, Portugal), Dr N. K. Barkov (Moscow, USSR), Dr A. Bertelsen (Aarhus, Denmark), Dr S. B. Blume (New York, NY, USA), Dr N. Bohacek (Zagreb, Yugoslavia), Dr A. Bracina Vieira (Lisbon, Portugal), Dr B. G. Burton-Bradley (Port Moresby, Papua New Guinea), Mrs K. Canavan (New Haven, CT, USA), Dr T. L. Chrusciel (Warsaw, Poland), Dr A. D. B. Clarke (Hull, England), Dr C. Climent (Cali, Colombia), Dr F. Cloutier (Paris, France), Dr P. H. Connell (London, England), Dr H. Davidian (Tehran, Islamic Republic of Iran), Dr K. C. Dube (Agra, India), Dr A. Dupont (Aarhus, Denmark), Dr J. Durell (Rockville, MD, USA), Dr M. Fakhr El-Islam (Kuwait), Dr W. Feindel (Montreal, Canada), Dr E. F. B. Forster (Accra, Ghana), Dr H. Gastaut (Marseille, France), Dr D. Goldberg (Manchester, England), Dr J. G. Gomez (Bogotá, Colombia), Dr J. Griffith Edwards (London, England), Dr H. Häfner (Mannheim, Federal Republic of Germany), Dr L. Hanzlicek (Prague, Czechoslovakia), Dr Hatai Chitanondh (Bangkok, Thailand), Dr Th. Hovaguimian (Geneva, Switzerland), Dr V. Hudolin (Zagreb, Yugoslavia), Dr G. Jeanneret (Geneva, Switzerland), Dr R. O. Jegede (Ibadan, Nigeria), Dr P. Kielholz (Basel, Switzerland), Dr L. Ladrido-Ignacio (Manila, the Philippines), Dr S. Lebovici (Paris, France), Dr P. V. Lemkau, (Baltimore, MD, USA), Dr Li Cong Pei (Beijing, China), Mr A. D. Loveday (WHO, Geneva, Switzerland), Mr D. A. Lowe (WHO, Geneva, Switzerland), Dr H. I. Maghazaji (Baghdad, Iraq), Dr J. Mardones (Santiago, Chile), Dr M. Masaaki Kato (Tokyo, Japan), Dr M. Mellergard (Copenhagen, Denmark), Dr P. V. Morozov (Moscow, USSR), Dr J. Martin Garcia (Madrid, Spain), Dr P. Munk-Jorgensen (Aarhus, Denmark), Dr Ö. Ödegaard (Oslo, Norway), Dr O. O. Ogunremi (Ilorin, Nigeria), Dr A. Okasha (Cairo, Egypt), Dr M. Öztürk (Ankara, Turkey), Dr K. J. Pataki-Schweizer (Boroko, Papua New Guinea), Dr C. Perris (Umeå, Sweden), Sir W. Refshauge (Canberra, Australia), Dr L. N. Robins (St Louis, MS, USA), Dr H. Rotondo Grimaldi (Lima, Peru), Dr M. Rutter (London, England), Dr S. Saxena, (New Delhi, India), Dr M. J. Sainsbury (Sydney, Australia), Dr L. F. Saugstad (Oslo, Norway), Dr H. Sell (WHO Regional Office for South East Asia, New Delhi, India), Dr N. Shinfuku (WHO Regional Office for the Western Pacific, Manila, Philippines), Dr Shi Yu-quan (Shanghai, China), Dr M. I. Soueif (Cairo, Egypt), Dr R. L. Spitzer (New York, NY, USA), Dr A. Stoller (Melbourne, Australia), Dr V. K. Varma (Chandigarh, India), Dr J.

Vymazal (Prague, Czechoslovakia), Dr I. Wald (Warsaw, Poland), Dr M. M. Weissman (New Haven, CT, USA), Dr N. N. Wig (WHO Regional Office for the Eastern Mediterranean, Alexandria, Egypt), Dr T. Yanagita (Kawasaki, Japan), Dr K. Zaimov (Sofia, Bulgaria), Dr D. von Zerssen (Munich, Federal Republic of Germany).

Index